Genetic Ties and the Family

Recent and Related Titles in Bioethics

Thomas H. Murray, consulting editor in bioethics

Genetic Ties and the Family

The Impact of Paternity Testing
on Parents and Children

Edited by
Mark A. Rothstein,
Thomas H. Murray,
Gregory E. Kaebnick,
and
Mary Anderlik Majumder

The Johns Hopkins University Press
Baltimore

The Johns Hopkins University Press
2715 North Charles Street
Baltimore, Maryland 21218-4363
MK www.press.jhu.edu

Library of Congress Cataloging-in-Publication Data

Genetic ties and the family : the impact of paternity testing on parents and children / edited by Mark A. Rothstein . . . [et al.].
    p.   cm.
Includes bibliographical references and index.
ISBN 0-8018-8193-5 (hardcover : alk. paper)
    1. Parent and child—United States. 2. Paternity—United States. 3. Parent and child (Law)—United States.
    [DNLM: 1. Parent-Child Relations—legislation & jurisprudence—United States. 2. Bioethical Issues—United States. 3. Paternity—United States. WS 33 AA1 G328 2006] I. Rothstein, Mark A.
    HQ755.85.G473 2006
    306.874′0973—dc22   2005003706

A catalog record for this book is available from the British Library.

In memory of our friend and colleague,
Dot Nelkin

Contents

Contributors

Lori B. Andrews, J.D., is Distinguished Professor of Law at Chicago-Kent College of Law; Director of the Institute for Science, Law and Technology at Illinois Institute of Technology; and Chairman of the Board at the Institute on Biotechnology and the Human Future. She received her B.A. (1975) and J.D. (1998) from Yale University.

Elizabeth Bartholet, J.D., is Morris Wasserstein Public Interest Professor of Law at Harvard Law School. She received her B.A. (1962) from Radcliffe College and LL.B. (1965) from Harvard University.

Jeffrey Blustein, Ph.D., is Professor of Bioethics at Albert Einstein College of Medicine of Yeshiva University; Faculty Associate at the Center for Bioethics at Columbia University; and Adjunct Associate Professor of Philosophy at Barnard College. He received his A.B. (1968) from the University of Minnesota and Ph.D. (1974) from Harvard University.

Nancy E. Dowd, J.D., Ph.D., is Chesterfield Smith Professor of Law and Associate Director of the Center on Children and the Law at the University of Florida. She received her B.A. (1971) from the University of Connecticut, M.A. (1973) and Ph.D. from the University of Illinois, and J.D. (1981) from Loyola University.

Michael Grossberg, Ph.D., is Professor of History and Adjunct Professor of Law at Indiana University and a Fellow of the Hastings Center. He received his B.A. (1972) from the University of California, Santa Barbara, and Ph.D. (1979) from Brandeis University.

Gregory E. Kaebnick, Ph.D., is an Associate for Philosophical Studies at the Hastings Center, in Garrison, New York. He received his B.A. (1986) from Swarthmore College and M.A. (1994) and Ph.D. (1998) from the University of Minnesota.

Mary Anderlik Majumder, J.D., Ph.D., is an Assistant Professor at the Center for Medical Ethics and Health Policy at Baylor College of Medicine. She received her B.A. (1985) from Bryn Mawr College, J.D. (1989) from Yale University, and Ph.D. (1997) from Rice University.

Thomas H. Murray, Ph.D., is the President of the Hastings Center, in Garrison, New York. He received his B.A. (1968) from Temple University and Ph.D. (1976) from Princeton University.

Dorothy Nelkin (deceased) was Professor of Sociology and Law at New York University. She received her B.A. (1954) from Cornell University.

Jeffrey A. Parness, J.D., is Professor of Law at Northern Illinois University College of Law. He received his B.A. (1968) from Colby College and J.D. (1974) from the University of Chicago.

Mark A. Rothstein, J.D., is Herbert F. Boehl Chair of Law and Medicine and Director of the Institute for Bioethics, Health Policy and Law at the University of Louisville. He received his B.A. (1970) from the University of Pittsburgh and J.D. (1973) from Georgetown University.

Diane Scott-Jones, Ph.D., is Professor of Psychology at Boston College. She received her B.S. (1971) and M.A. (1972) from Appalachian State University and Ph.D. (1979) from the University of North Carolina.

Dan Wulff, Ph.D., is Associate Professor and Co-Director of the Family Therapy Program at Kent School of Social Work, University of Louisville. He received his B.S. (1976) from Iowa State University, M.S.W. (1976) from the University of Iowa, and Ph.D. (1994) from Iowa State University.

Preface

Perhaps no grouping of individuals is as important in our society as the family. In recent years, the characterization of the family unit has been affected by advances in genetics, which have greatly increased the amount and accuracy of biological information about people. DNA-based identity testing is capable of quickly, inexpensively, and accurately establishing the presence or absence of biological relationships among people in intimate familial relationships. Genetic identity testing has had many beneficial and humanitarian applications, such as reuniting war orphans with grandparents and other relatives and confirming disputed parentage. Genetic testing also has helped to undermine or even disestablish existing family relationships, often causing great emotional pain to children and parents alike.

As demonstrated by adoption and artificial reproductive technologies, a genetic or biological relationship is not coextensive with a family relationship. Yet, biological relatedness traditionally has been the starting point for legal conceptions of the family, with important implications for child custody, child support, heirship, and other matters. In a new scientific era in which biological relationships can be established with virtual certainty, what legal and social import should be given to such information? In other words, how should society resolve the tension between biological and social notions of the family?

To address these and related questions, we assembled a group of experts from a variety of disciplines, including bioethics, history, law, pediatrics, philosophy, psychology, social work, and sociology. Our research was supported by a grant from the National Human Genome Research Institute of the National Institutes of Health. We held three workshops at the Hastings Center and sponsored a public conference in New Orleans, on March 27 and 28, 2003, to explore these issues. Many of the chapters in this volume had their origins in presentations at these meetings. Other aspects of our research, including a survey of genetic testing laboratories, were separately published in various journals.

We would like to acknowledge the assistance of the following experts who participated in our workshops or supplied us with valuable information: Adrienne Asch, Caroline Caskey, Christi Goodman, Erik Parens, Mary Lyndon Shanley, and Elizaveta Veikher. We would also like to recognize Carrie Besser for her research and citation checking and Jodi Fernandez and Sue Rose for their excellent work in preparing the manuscript for publication.

Introduction: The Many-Stranded Tapestry of Parenthood

Gregory E. Kaebnick, Ph.D., and
Thomas H. Murray, Ph.D.

Biomedical technology is forcing us to rethink subjects that may seem remote from medicine and science. The meaning of life, a person's capacity to make decisions about her life, the nature of selfhood, even the nature of nature itself, have all been put on the table for fresh discussion. One of the threads woven into the tapestry of images and narratives that shape and represent human family life—and one that has received less attention than it deserves—is the nature of parenthood.

Perhaps everybody who comes home from the hospital with a newborn looks for traits that show the child's pedigree. Certainly every grandparent who visits the next week clucks over some claimed resemblance, no matter how difficult it is for others to see. But what do such biological connections really signify? What is the place of biology in parenthood? It might amount to nothing of any genuine importance, at least when compared with what parents ought to *do* for their children—providing and protecting, nourishing and guiding. But it is sometimes taken to signify much more: a biological connection is sometimes thought to be *constitutive*—partially or in whole—of the parental relationship. Or, striking a course somewhere between these two extremes, the biological connection might be legitimately valued by some parents and children as a vital strand within the particular narrative they will share as children and parents but might be altogether missing in other families—with no damage or loss to the relationship.

These questions have always been with us, but they have recently acquired a new and sometimes chilling urgency. DNA testing can now reliably show whether the biological relationship exists, allowing parents, children, and others to conclusively resolve questions that previously could not be answered with precision. British and American law has long held that a biological relationship between a child and the husband of the child's mother must almost always be assumed to exist. According to the "marital presumption" (also known as the "presumption of legitimacy"), a child born to a woman within a marriage is irrebuttably presumed to be the biological child of the woman's husband, unless he was absent, impotent, or sterile. To many observers, the presumption seems antiquated. Why settle for a presumption if science can reveal the facts?

Given this new ability, what we decide about the place of biology in parenthood leads to another question: what should people be able to do when they learn something new about their biological and parental relationships? And, further, should there be restraints on when or how such information can be learned? In the great majority of cases, it is paternity that is at issue (reasonably reliable empirical indicators of genetic motherhood having long been available). Sometimes, genetic testing conducted for other reasons functions indirectly as paternity testing. In one case, a man discovered he was not the biological father of a child when the child was diagnosed with cystic fibrosis (a recessive disorder that must be inherited from both parents) and the man learned he did not carry the cystic fibrosis mutation. But in a growing number of cases, genetic testing is conducted purely to assess paternity. It may be sought by a man with the possible goal either of terminating a parental relationship, with its attendant responsibilities, or of asserting his right to establish a parental relationship. It may be sought by the child's mother either to impose parental responsibilities on a man or to deny parental rights to a man. Finally, it may be sought by others—the children, relatives, distant descendants, child support enforcement agencies—for a variety of reasons: to determine parental responsibilities, to influence family relationships, to learn something medically useful, to establish lines of descent or inheritance, or simply out of curiosity.

New technologies seem often to be followed, conveniently enough, by the discovery of human desires to which those technologies can respond. In the opening chapter of this volume, the late sociologist Dorothy Nelkin argues that the availability of a genetic test for paternity has reinforced the tendency to see biology as the basis of parenthood. Strands in Western culture have long ascribed a special significance to "blood ties" and "bloodlines," but, as Nelkin sees it, those ties are now said to be of overriding importance. Nelkin points to a variety of possible causes: promotions by the companies that offer the tests, amplification of their message by the media, a widespread belief that contemporary family relationships need more certainty and stability, and the broad acceptance of a "genetic essentialism," according to which DNA is the "invisible but fundamental basis of human identity, explaining our place in the world, our behavior, our fate—and our proper social relationships." The very label "paternity test" suggests that the test assesses not merely a genetic relationship but also a full paternal relationship—*fatherhood*. If fatherhood flows fully and completely from a genetic relationship, then "misattributed paternity" implies the complete absence of fatherhood. When identifying the father, not only is the marital presumption no longer necessary, it scarcely feels possible—at best a quaint historical anachronism.

Nelkin quotes an article in the *New York Times* as saying that genetic paternity testing "hit the popular marketplace" in the late 1990s (Belluck 1997). According to the American Association of Blood Banks, which accredits most of the labs offering genetic testing, 76,000 paternity tests were conducted in 1988, 247,000 in 1998, and 280,000 in 1999. An industry worth around $100 million, according to some press reports, sprang into being to sell genetic testing services. Billboards plugging the services cropped up along highways, displaying such messages as "who's the father?" and "is his mother a liar?" Web sites reassured visitors that a court order is usually not required to permit a paternity test and that "accurate paternity testing can be performed when the mother is not available." Television talk shows introduced paternity testing into their family fun: not only is Mandy sleeping with Mark's best friend, but Matt is not Mark's son, and a DNA test will prove it on-air. Fathers' rights groups have embraced paternity testing as a way of protecting "duped dads" from "paternity fraud"; their Web sites warn that men are in great danger of being "deceived, scammed, and hustled" into making child support payments for another man's child.

All this agitation in favor of paternity testing has begun to wrest American law away from the marital presumption. The law concerning paternity testing is in disarray and in flux, as Mary Anderlik Majumder notes in chapter 10 of this volume. Federal law tends to encourage the use of genetic testing to establish paternity, chiefly to increase the likelihood that fathers who deny that they owe child support can be forced to pay it. State law tends to permit the use of genetic testing to establish paternity but not to challenge paternity (Ohio H.B. 242, 1999, enacted July 27, 2000). Yet the states vary considerably in their approach to genetic testing, and an increasing number are introducing and approving legislation to facilitate use of genetic paternity testing in court. Some commentators believe that, if the testing fully establishes itself in society, divorce lawyers could end up routinely recommending that their clients obtain genetic paternity testing.

For the last several years, we at the Hastings Center have been collaborating with Mark Rothstein and Mary Anderlik Majumder, at the University of Louisville's Institute for Bioethics, Health Policy and Law, to study this issue. In the course of a project funded by the National Institutes of Health and led by Rothstein and Thomas Murray, we have invited people in the areas of law, child psychology, family counseling, history, and philosophy and from the genetic paternity testing industry to a series of meetings at the Hastings Center to discuss and develop policy for the field. First, we sought to develop a conceptual overview of the family. We asked, what do *parenthood* and *family* mean? What are the rights and responsibilities of parents? How can we assess the significance of children's interests? And how does a genetic relationship between parent and child bear on all of these things? From this starting point we turned to the social context in which paternity testing is used. We asked about the consequences for families and children of the different ways genetic paternity testing can be used. Finally, we brought the conceptual and empirical work to bear on the current policy framework for paternity testing, both the regulation of the laboratories that offer the tests and the state law stipulating the use that parents may make of the tests.

This book is a product of that work, and the authors were participants in those meetings. The first part of the book explores the philosophical and social background. Nelkin's opening chapter on the media blitz about paternity testing is an entry point into the debate over genetic paternity testing. Nelkin suggests that the media have helped foment what they purport only to witness and respond to—namely, the growing popular interest in and felt need for paternity testing. Chapters 2 through 6 all explore the significance of parenthood, although from different perspectives, using different tools, and with somewhat different concerns foremost. In chapter 2, Murray offers an analysis of the cultural meanings and models of parenthood. What is fundamental to parenthood, he argues, is that it is a "rearing relationship," understanding this as a many-stranded connection between child and adult. The rights and responsibilities that characterize the relationship, he continues, are best understood on the model of what he calls *mutualism,* meaning that the relationship promotes the flourishing of both parents and children. The genetic link between parent and child can be an important part of that relationship—but need not be.

In chapter 3, philosopher Jeffrey Blustein asks about the bases of parental obligations and rights and whether an account of them provides any restrictions on what genetic paternity testing may be used to argue for. A biological relationship with a child typically leads to obligations to the child: someone who has brought a child into the world must see that the child is well cared for. But a biological relationship is not the only way of incurring that obligation, Blustein argues, and it does not automatically give a man the right to establish something more. A man who is not biologically related to a child but has nonetheless acted as a father cannot simply walk away from the relationship or be pushed aside.

Chapters 4 and 5 take up the social context. First, psychologist Diane Scott-Jones considers what parenthood means for children's development. She argues that the social and psychological aspects of fathering are important for children and should be promoted and protected, even if they cannot all be enforced, and that a genetic tie is not essential for filling this role. Discovering that a presumed genetic tie does not exist can be difficult, for children as well as fathers, but whether and how it is difficult will vary depending both on the child's developmental level and on many, complex aspects of family relationships.

The complexity of families is underscored by Dan Wulff, a family counselor and professor of social work. "All general understandings of families and their patterns of behavior ought to be held 'lightly,'" writes Wulff. When counselors think about the effects of paternity testing on any given family, they should be informed by what they have seen or learned about other families, but they should always be ready to find something new, given cultural variation in beliefs about the family, ongoing change within cultures, and the infinite complexity of individuals.

In chapter 6, concluding the first part of the book, law professor Nancy Dowd offers an agenda for changing the social context to give women and men equal standing in the family. Fatherhood should be defined by what fathers *do* instead of by what they are, says Dowd, and the doing that is critical is nurture. Making nurture central to fatherhood requires socioeconomic change: if fathers continue to be seen as the primary economic support of children, then they will continue to be seen *primarily as* economic support, and egalitarian, cooperative parenting will be unachievable.

The second part of the book addresses the law. Historian Michael Grossberg, launching the discussion with a review of the legal history, finds that genetic paternity testing perpetuates centuries-old tensions in the laws concerning the nature of parenthood and the responsibilities that attach to fatherhood. Yet this history also shows the possibility of broad transformation even in a fundamental institution such as the family. An understanding of the long-standing tensions underlying paternity testing, argues Grossberg, can help illuminate the consequences of transformations, both those in our history and those we confront in the near future.

Chapters 8 and 9 offer prescriptions for change. Law professor Elizabeth Bartholet accepts as a premise what Blustein and others have argued, that a genetic relationship does not alone establish parenthood and that a child-parent relationship, once created, should not be terminated solely on the grounds that a genetic relationship has been disproved. Bartholet's recommended "core principles" would ensure that, in determining parentage, society views biology as a limited factor, outweighed by the child's interests. Some "related rules of the road" would help ensure stable, nurturing families.

Law professor Jeffrey Parness argues that the current institutional mechanisms for selecting parents treat men unfairly. Women nearly always enjoy at least an opportunity to establish parental rights with a child to whom they are genetically related; men do not. Parness's solution is to reform birth certificate laws to promote "early, complete, accurate, informed, and conclusive legal paternity designations."

In chapter 10, Mary Anderlik Majumder explores the efforts already under way to reform and clarify paternity law. She finds rapid change but "little evidence of consensus." Her review of recent court decisions and state actions reveals a spectrum of views about the significance of a genetic relationship, with most holding that genetics is relevant, sometimes even important, but not decisive, and many relying heavily on what they consider to be the best interests of the child.

Lori Andrews, a legal scholar who has written widely on new reproductive technologies, argues in chapter 11 that those who look to biology to determine parentage are at odds with the dominant trends in case law and statute for identifying the parents of children created through assisted reproduction—egg and sperm donation, surrogate motherhood, and posthumous use of a man's sperm. In these contexts, parentage is likely to be settled not by genetic relationship but by the intent to bring children into the world and raise them.

Andrews concludes that not only the use of genetic paternity testing but even mere access to it warrants legal constraint.

In the final chapter, Mark Rothstein draws from the preceding analyses and proposals to develop a set of recommendations for amending the Uniform Parentage Act of 2000, a model law drafted by the National Conference of Commissioners on Uniform State Laws. He also reviews and analyzes a range of policy options for regulating the laboratories that offer genetic paternity testing.

In this volume, none of the authors defends the marital presumption, at least as it has traditionally been articulated, but all defend or accept the presumption's unarticulated core principle—that a family is something people establish, not something that biological relationship establishes for them. As traditionally articulated, the marital presumption does not question the view that parenthood rests on a biological relationship, and indeed the presumption's other name, the "presumption of legitimacy," suggests that a biological relationship is the appropriate template. But the law's overriding goal was to assure that the financial responsibility for children did not fall to the state. The presumption that children born to married couples are the biological offspring of the husband is a fiction embraced to pursue this goal. The marital presumption could always fly in the face of the biological facts, even when they were very widely known: everybody in the shire might know that the son was not biologically related to the father. The marital presumption, with its many defects, nonetheless contains one core insight worth preserving: even without a genetic connection, a family is possible. This central point is recast by Blustein as one of the presumptive principles of parental obligations, it recurs throughout this book in various formulations, and it informs the policy recommendations at the end.

Very likely, even if the parentage system were reformed and all of the recommendations discussed here adopted, the system would not always prevent parents from evading their responsibilities, denying other parents their parental rights, and disrupting children's lives, as Rothstein notes toward the end of the book. Parents could still sometimes game the system. Yet one might hope that reform of the parentage system would have the converse effect of the arrival of genetic testing. Nelkin tells us that genetic testing and the media attention surrounding it (along with genetic science in general) have reinvigorated the traditional view that parenthood is fundamentally about biology. Yet as Grossberg, Murray, Wulff, and Scott-Jones remind us, there is another long-established, honorable, and insightful view about parenthood, according to which parenthood is fundamentally a *personal* relationship—a social and psychological phenomenon that emphasizes nurture, commitment, and support. Perhaps a reformed parentage system could, by explaining and defending this view, not merely enforce it but reinforce it and pull public opinion in its train.

Murray describes the relationship between parent and child as a tapestry, a many-stranded phenomenon, woven by both parties and incorporating and meeting the moral and developmental needs of both. Wulff adds that this relationship is diverse and variable. So understood, parenthood can certainly not be reduced to the genetic tie, nor is the genetic tie even an essential part of it. Yet the genetic tie could still be one of its strands. In various ways, sometimes in dramatically different ways, all the contributors to this volume may end up endorsing this view. At one end of the spectrum, Dowd argues that the personal relationship provides the only appropriate basis for determinations of parentage and that men should be parents only when they fully share in the nurturing that children require, but she adds that children can benefit from knowing their genetic relationships. At the other end, Parness argues that a genetic relationship should come with an opportunity to establish a personal relationship and that, for men, this opportunity needs promotion and protection. In some families, the genetic tie is a component of the tapestry that family members weave and, indeed, a part of it that they value. It can be missing from other stories without any loss—other strands could replace it. If the consensus in this volume is correct, the genetic tie is not the foundation of the family.

BIBLIOGRAPHY

Belluck, P. 1997. Paternity testing for fun and profit. *New York Times,* 3 August.
Egerton B. 1999. DNA tests don't let dads off the hook: Man supports sons not biologically his. *Dallas Morning News,* 31 October.
Lewin, T. 2001. In genetic testing for paternity, law often lags behind science. *New York Times,* 11 March.
Michael H. v. Gerald D. 1989. 491 U.S. 110, 124.

Part I / Family Values

The Shifting Ground of the Parent-Child Relationship

CHAPTER ONE

Paternity Palaver in the Media

Selling Identity Tests

Dorothy Nelkin

The *Montel Williams Show,* a prime-time television talk show, featured a divorced couple squabbling over custody arrangements for their child. The man had provided child support and maintained continued contact with the boy, suggesting his real emotional commitment. But his former wife claimed that he was not, in fact, the child's "real"—that is, "biological"—father. The man, plagued with suspicion, allowed the talk-show host to order a DNA test. The test results, announced on-air, provided the proof that his former wife was right: he was not the biological dad. The host then declared that this man "now has to de-bond with a baby he believed to be his" (*Montel Williams Show* 1997).

This is one of the many talk shows, soap operas, late-night dramas, tabloid stories, advice columns, Internet messages, and news reports that are capitalizing on the entertainment value—the titillation and trauma—of the cuckolded husbands and troubled families who are buying into DNA identity tests. There are amazing stories about strange cases: a ten-year-old girl whose aborted fetus was tested so that prosecutors could prove incest; a family of seven children in their forties who discovered through tests that they had three different fathers; a woman with seven brothers who were tested to discover which one was father to her child. The media stories—purportedly real-life dramas—are selected and embellished for popular consumption. As Allen Gelb, a self-identified immunohematologist who presents DNA results on many television talk shows and also testifies in court, observed, "The more devastating the news, the better the ratings" (quoted in Taylor 2000).

It is important to track such media coverage, for repeated stories in the media provide insight into popular perceptions and social anxieties. Media narratives also shape public attitudes. The selection and presentation of events, the stories and interpretations, can influence social morals, consumer demands, and intimate relationships as well as legal decisions and public policies (Nelkin 1994). Strikingly preoccupied with paternity testing, the media are building on and reinforcing anxieties about changing family relationships. Their stories and reports are fueling the demand for DNA identification tests and promoting a burgeoning business by amplifying the marketing strategies of DNA testing firms.

There are many uses of DNA identity tests, the most common being the identification of suspected criminals. Identity tests are also used, however, by immigration officials as a means to verify claimed relationships. They have been used to identify lost or kidnapped children, accident victims, victims of military atrocities, soldiers who fathered "war babies," and Alzheimer's wanderers. DNA tests were used in Bosnia to identify the remains in unmarked graves, in Argentina to identify the children of the "disappeared," and in New York City to identify the remains of people who were killed and often burned beyond recognition at the World Trade Center on September 11, 2001. They are also useful to identify skeletal remains for historical and archaeological research and for studies of ancient migration patterns.

Media interest, however, has focused a great deal of attention on the use of DNA tests to verify paternity. Tabloids pursue cases of paternity fraud: "Who's the daddy?" Soap operas and television dramas revolve around the tensions and uncertainties of paternity—uncertainties to be resolved by genetic tests. Television talk shows feature "live" paternity testing, as on the *Montel Williams Show*. The paternity struggles of celebrities, from Thomas Jefferson to Bill Cosby, from Yves Montand to Hollywood producer Steve Bing, are displayed in the news. Advice columnists advise their readers to resolve their suspicions by getting tested. Highway billboards attract commuters to genetic testing firms. Especially important are the growing number of Web sites that are providing information, advertisements, and promotional discussions about the value of paternity testing. The public is bombarded with paternity palaver.

Sorting through this media blitz, I found three repeated claims:

- "Real" relationships depend on shared DNA.
- Infidelity and paternity fraud are so rampant that there are real reasons for suspicion.
- There is a burning need—on both economic and emotional grounds—to know the biological truth.

The message conveyed is that DNA tests are commercially available to resolve troubling uncertainties by revealing biological truth.

The Marketing of DNA Testing

The media coverage of paternity testing reflects the interests of a burgeoning and aggressive genetic testing industry seeking to expand its market. The media, perhaps unwittingly, are building their stories on industry advertising, amplifying promotional messages, and directly serving corporate goals.

Taxicabs in New York City carry on their roofs an advertisement—"Call 1-800-DNA-Type." A billboard on a Baltimore expressway displays a very pregnant version of the Mona Lisa with her enigmatic smile: "Who's the daddy?" The billboard provides the phone number of the laboratory that offers DNA paternity tests (Spector 1999).

This laboratory, Identigene, was founded in 1993 by Caroline Caskey, daughter of geneticist Tom Caskey, the president and CEO of Cogene Biotech Ventures. She uses DNA testing to verify the paternity relationships of her clients. She describes the company's ads as intended to "bang you over the head and make you take notice." They have, indeed, helped her to expand her DNA testing business: "We are creating a new market" (Mirabella 1997). Identigene's Web site includes a "guess the father" game that displays pictures of a beaming baby and three potential dads. If you click on the correct face, you are told "lucky guess" and then informed that many children, in fact, do not look like their parents. The point is that there is much room for doubt, and doubt can be easily dispelled by a DNA test. Identigene's "is she cheating?" messages have helped to create "a massive new client base" for the testing industry, based on suspicions of infidelity. Indeed, paternity laboratories get phone calls and visits every day from suspicious men who see genetic identity testing as a way to resolve their uncertainties about the fidelity of their wives.

Many paternity testing companies are mail-order operations based on the Internet. A Google search in 2003 revealed 330 Web sites for paternity testing services. A company called Genetic Identity advertises services that, it claims, are affordable, friendly, accurate, expert (only Ph.D. scientists), fast (three to five days), and so competent that the company gives a money-back guarantee (though it is not quite clear what is guaranteed). Another company, DNA Virtual, opens its Web site with the tag line "The Power to Solve" (though it is not quite clear what is to be solved).

Also promoted on the Internet are home testing kits. The Web site www.
D-FWMall.com offers "swift response" DNA home-collection kits. The DNA
Testing Centre, Inc., informs its clients that they can use cigarette butts, chewed
gum, Q-Tips, electric razor debris, used condoms, or plucked hair. Clients are
to send the samples or swabs to the lab by mail, and the results will be returned
within seven business days. Home tests are also promoted: easy to do in the
comfort of your own home by simply wiping a cotton swab inside the mouths
of father and child and mailing in the sample.

The wide appeal of these Web sites is suggested by an advertising list on
a "pay for performance" site called www.goto.com (or www.overture.com),
which includes more than fifty paternity testing companies. The companies
pay more than $2.10 per click (or hit) to hold the top place on the list. This
cost per hit is relatively high, indicating its value in directing targeted customers to the company sites. For example, when one types the word *cars* into
www.goto.com, the top advertiser that comes up pays only forty cents per
click, significantly less than the bid of the paternity testing companies.

Meanwhile, media stories—catering to the backlash against demands for
child support, to anxiety and suspicion, or to the titillating effect of "messy
unmentionables"—are providing free advertising. They are, in effect, amplifying the marketing messages of the paternity testing firms.

In pursuit of interesting stories, journalists sometimes write about specific
companies and their most newsworthy cases. The *Baltimore Sun* describes the
work of the Baltimore-based RH Laboratory. Tests at this lab have reunited
a kidnapped child with his parents, resolved the anxiety of a woman who
feared that her pregnancy had resulted from a rape, and relieved the uncertainty of a young couple who suspected they might be half siblings (Mirabella
1997).

The *Tennessean* describes the daily job of a lab technician at Lifecodes who
has opened packages containing unlaundered underpants. The suspicious
sender wants to find out whether his sweetheart's DNA is commingled with a
third party's. The technician also takes samples from tampons, condoms, and
used hankies. Her stories, writes the reporter, are very popular at dinner parties (Ferguson 2001).

Through their repeated narratives, journalists have normalized the practice
of going for DNA tests: finding out "who's the father" appears as the most important issue around. The *New York Times* writes, for example, that "paternity

testing is no longer the surreptitiously shameful province of Family Court, of the spurned, blackmailing mistress. It has hit the popular marketplace" (Belluck 1997). "Everybody's doing it," screams the header to this article. The *Augusta Chronicle* announces "a secret that's fast getting out . . . DNA tests aren't just for the O. J. Simpsons of the world" (Associated Press 1997). The *Tennessean* notes the urgency of the issue, quoting an official from Genetic Technologies, Inc.: "We've had investigators go into motels, pay off the house-keepers and get sheets . . . You'd be amazed at what people will resort to" (Ferguson 2001).

Advice columnists, who are often asked about testing, even provide the names of companies that will clear up doubts about paternity. Ann Landers wrote that, if a man questions the paternity of a child, a DNA test can be very valuable. "You need to know, once and for all, whether you are the child's father" (Landers 2000). Company ads and the media conduits employ several arguments to attract clients to their services: they define "real" relationships as based on shared DNA, they seek to cultivate suspicion, and they insist on the deep economic and emotional need to know the biological truth.

"Real" Relationships Are Based on Shared DNA

On the *Montel Williams Show,* shared genes were of overriding importance in defining the "real" family. Thus when the paternity test revealed that the father had no biological connection to a child he thought his own, the information defined the man as outside the family, despite his long-standing emotional and social commitment. He became a "biological stranger." He had to "de-bond."

In a story about the reunion of a disrupted and long-separated family, the Delta Airlines magazine, *Sky,* describes "genetic suction." "There must be some deep magnetism well below consciousness that draws related people together—something to do with genetic suction" (Fulghum 1995, 35).

The film *The Deep End of the Ocean* is about a ten-year-old boy who was kidnapped as an infant and adopted by a caring family. He is then "restored" to his "real"—that is, biological—family. Though the boy does not remember his biological family, the message is that his genetic ties are the immutable and irrefutable link to his legitimacy as a person. This is an archetypal narrative, one that is repeated in numerous baby-switching and adoption stories; the "real" family is bound together less by history, tradition, or common experience than by shared DNA. "Real" parents are those who contribute gametes, because "real" connections depend on shared DNA. This is the premise underlying the explosion of paternity testing and the willing and uncritical popular acceptance of this practice, which, I will suggest, is not necessarily so benign.

This idea, that the only real relationships are biologically based, reflects the growing belief in "genetic essentialism" since the 1980s, as the gene has become a cultural icon (Nelkin and Lindee 1995). In both the language of scientists and the parables of popular culture, DNA has become an invisible but fundamental basis of human identity, explaining our place in the world, our behavior, our fate—and our proper social relationships.

But the critical importance of biological relationships also fits well with traditional concepts of the family in American and Western cultures (Finkler 2001; Schneider 1968). Common aphorisms about "blood lines" and "blood ties" and the pervasive belief that "blood is thicker than water," as well as classic stories such as *Oliver Twist,* have long built on the importance of genetic identity. We are raised with the idea that shared genes are stronger than emotional connections, social commitment, or shared experience. Families that operate outside this biological model—for example, those with illegitimate or adopted children—must often deal with the social assessment that they are inauthentic, not quite "real." Repeated stories about the tragic fate of stepchildren or the needs of adoptees to find their "real" parents express the cultural expectation that real families are based on ties of blood.

The popular preoccupation with genetic connections is related in part to concerns about recent changes in family life. Genes seem to offer an apparently solid basis for human connections at a time when the status of the family as a troubled institution is well entrenched in popular and political culture. Threatened by feminism, divorce, working mothers, gay and lesbian partnerships, and the complex arrangements enabled by reproductive technologies, the family seems to be in a state of crisis (Nelkin and Lindee 1995). Particularly important for our consideration of paternity palaver are the changes in the family that have shifted the relative status of men and women and fostered a sense of male victimization. A fathers' rights movement expresses resentment about the pursuit of "deadbeat dads" and a resistance to court decisions that seem to favor moms. Pervading many families is an aura of suspicion and mistrust—and this is deliberately cultivated by paternity testing firms.

Cultivating Suspicion

Lionel Tiger, in his best-selling book *The Decline of Males* (1999), writes about the confidence and power of women and the eroding confidence of men. Cultivating suspicion is easy among men who feel marginalized by changes in the traditional relationships between men and women. Resentment is fostered in the popular press through portrayals of men who are "nagged by doubts."

A highway billboard that advertises a genetic testing laboratory pictures a baby with a Pinocchio nose: "Is his mother a liar?" Another ad, taking off on *Star Wars,* reads, "Luke, I am your father . . . uh, I think" (Spector 1999). The slogan of the testing company Identigene is "peace of mind through DNA testing" (Identigene 2005)—though the truth may yield anything but. The Web site of the Phoenix-based company, Forensex Laboratories Corporation, www.sementest.com, tells potential customers to send in garments that might contain semen stains, and promises that results will be promptly returned by phone or mail: "Send us your dirty panties."

Such media reports seem to be sounding an alarm. They are full of statistics showing that infidelity is rampant. According to various widely repeated media estimates, as many as 5 to 20 percent of people in the United States are wrong about their paternity. And as many as 30 percent of the men who take paternity tests find that their suspicions were warranted, for the children they are supporting are in fact unrelated to them (Rogers 2000). Their wives have cheated. These men are described in the media and especially in Internet communications as innocent victims, suckers, cuckolded, betrayed, deceived, and duped. They have been subjected to indignity, distress, and humiliation. The number of men so victimized is described on Web sites as "astounding," "alarming." "Are you one of the 30 percent?" There is good reason, these data suggest, for suspicion (Citizens against Paternity Fraud 2001).

Horror stories in the media compound suspicion and mistrust. Women are engaged in "monstrous infidelity." Men, once "deadbeat dads," are now "duped dads" (E. Goodman 2001). They are triple victims: of infidelity, child support, and the loss of their children. A repeatedly reported story of victimization is the case of Morgan Wise, a divorced Texan, who took a paternity test when one of his four children developed cystic fibrosis, a genetic disease that, to his knowledge, was not in his family. Wise was tested to find out whether he was a cystic fibrosis carrier, but instead he discovered that three of the children he had supported as his own were, in fact, not biologically related to him. His relationship with his children unraveled. He tried to stop paying child support, but the court refused to let him off. The court also suspended his visitation rights (Kelleher 2001).

Similar victimization of fathers, according to media reports, is happening throughout the country. It is so rampant that some lawyers recommend advising every man who is getting a divorce to get paternity testing. "Now it seems like it could be malpractice not to warn them" (Lewin 2001).

In media stories, men have been especially victimized by child support laws. The courts, basing their decisions on a long commitment to protect the best interests of the child, have for the most part been unwilling to remove the obligation for child support on the basis of paternity tests. Many reporters are sympathetic to men whose demands are turned down, portraying them as "victims" who are treated unfairly. Even wrongly convicted prisoners have a better fate. Criminals are exonerated on the basis of DNA tests; why not dads? (Gumbel 2001). One seldom finds references these days to "deadbeat dads." The focus has shifted. The real problem seems to be "paternity fraud."

New lobbying groups with such names as Citizens against Paternity Fraud convey the need for suspicion. Their members, widely dispersed, communicate through the Internet. The Web site www.PaternityFraud.com portrays Uncle Sam, surrounded by dollar signs, pointing his finger at the viewer: "I'll get you for being a Dad." These groups are part of the fathers' rights movement, which is demanding "parental equality." Members of Fathers for Equal Rights complain that they see guys freed from prison every day through DNA testing, but fathers seem to have fewer rights.

The widely promulgated theories of sociobiology and evolutionary psychology have helped to fuel suspicion by suggesting that "infidelity is in the genes." Infidelity is functional and, therefore, natural. David Barash and Judith Lipton, in a popular book, *The Myth of Monogamy: Fidelity and Infidelity in Animals and People* (2001), claim that infidelity is in the genes of almost every animal species including *Homo sapiens*. Featured in nearly a hundred television, radio, and magazine reports, they claim that people are totally fascinated with adultery because everyone has been affected by it or has thought about it. "The evidence is really undeniable, that monogamy among animals is more myth than reality."

Women as well as men gain from multiple sex partners, writes Tom Birkhead in his book *Promiscuity* (2000). Females with multiple partners have had an evolutionary advantage because this assures protection of their children. These theories legitimate suspicion. There are good science-based reasons for men to suspect their women, writes *New York Times* science editor Nicholas Wade: "The next time you look over a cradle into those innocent eyes and half formed smile, remember the old saying: 'Mother's baby, father's maybe'" (Wade 2001). In this context, there seems to be a burning need to know the truth.

The Need to Know the Biological "Truth"

> Whose child is this? A question that tugs at the heartstrings and the purse strings.
> —ASSOCIATED PRESS 1997

The public is deluged with corporate messages and media stories suggesting there is a burning need to know the biological truth about identity. The reason? First and foremost is the issue of money—the negotiation of child support or the verification of inheritance claims. Second is the quest for emotional wholeness—the belief that revealing genetic relationships will verify who we are and what we are. DNA testing also satisfies curiosity; it is part of the celebrity fascination, a way to know the truth about famous people.

The Purse Strings

The *Augusta Chronicle* tells the story of a family that received a six-figure insurance settlement when their seventeen-year-old boy died in a car crash. The mother's first husband showed up, wanting his share of the money, but the mother insisted that another man, whom she later married, was the real dad. A DNA test proved she was right (Associated Press 1997). But most media stories focus on avoiding child support. They are stories of victimized fathers, the "duped dads" who need to know the truth to protect their assets.

During the 1990s, laws in many states forced fathers ("deadbeat dads") who had not paid child support to pay up. Resentment of these laws has motivated many men to wonder whether the children they are supporting are, in fact, biologically related to them. The biological truth, they believe, will put an end to their victimization. The refusal of many courts to buy their argument is described in the media and especially on Web sites as unfair. In the context of paternity fraud, men need to know the truth to protect their deepest interests. "Save a life (yours) by getting your DNA paternity test done today. Accused Dads deserve to know the truth." "The mother can refuse to let you see the children, come after your cash and assets and use the law to rob you blind."

Paternity fraud is "financial rape." Or paternity fraud is an "international epidemic" (Smith 2001). The Web site www.Divorcenet.com posts messages on paternity issues. Most messages are about money, about the victimization of fathers obliged to support children even though they are not the biological father. Should a man have to continue paying child support when he is not the biological father?

The media are also attracted to cases of extortion that involve the use of paternity tests, especially when they involve entertainment figures or other high-profile people. Bill Cosby entertained the public with his own real-life sit-com when Autumn Jackson claimed to be his illegitimate daughter and demanded $40 million to keep the story out of the tabloids. Cosby denied the claim and agreed to be tested, and Jackson was convicted of extortion (Zoglin and Faltermayer 1997).

French actor Yves Montand died in 1991, just before he was to testify against a woman who claimed to be his daughter. The woman wanted a share of his fortune. Montand, who refused to have a DNA test when alive, was disinterred for testing. There was no match (Starnes 1998). Journalists cover such DNA tests as a way to "root out gold-diggers" who try to make money on false paternity claims. Exhumation is increasingly common as a means to resolve inheritance disputes—the claims of contested wills or the right to the Social Security benefits of deceased relatives.

The Heartstrings

GeneLink, a New Jersey firm, markets a kit enabling funeral directors, for a sizeable fee, to retrieve DNA from the deceased. This company caters to people who will pay to save the genes of their loved ones so they can clarify or resolve troubling ambiguities about their genetic roots.

Media stories suggest that establishing the truth about genetic connections is essential for one's sense of identity and emotional wholeness. The message that genes are the basis of identity frequently appears in adoption narratives. For example, a writer who was adopted at birth describes in *Parenting* magazine his desperate search for his biological parents. Feeling neither real nor whole, he writes about his "unquenchable thirst" for his roots. When the adoption agency finally locates his mother, he writes, "I sensed a kind of completion for the first time in my life" (Weizel 1991, 90).

Critics of adoption practices call adoption a pathology that "counters the dictates of nature." They refer to adoptees as amputees, describing them as troubled, with impaired "identity formation." *Psychology Today* explored the problem of "genealogical bewilderment," a sense that lack of information about genetic relationships prevents the forming of a sense of self (Kaye 1980). Numerous adoption advice books describe the "quest for wholeness" and the "quest for roots," suggesting that without identifying her real—that is, biological—parents, a person cannot be complete or fulfilled.

The widely accepted practice of sperm donation—a common source of financial support and tuition for medical students—has gone on for years under conditions of anonymity. But the genetic age, with its assumptions about the importance of genetic identity, has generated disputes over the rights of sperm donors and their children to have access to information about their kin. People conceived through donor insemination ("remote father conception") have organized to express their right to know their genetic origins. "We need the roadmap of our genetic blueprint." "I was conceived like pigs are, with no rights to know my genetic heritage" (Norton 2000).

The children of sperm donors communicate with one another mainly through electronic mailing lists such as www.egroups.com/community/ spermdonors. The Donor Conception Network publicizes their "plight" and helps them gain access to their genetic heritage by searching for biological fathers. Several countries have sperm donor registries through which offspring can trace their biological fathers. In the United States, a growing number of sperm banks offer a voluntary system of donor identification release in which donors agree that their offspring will be able to obtain information on how to contact them.

Reflected in these changes is the belief that establishing DNA identity— that is, verifying biological relationships—meets a deep emotional need. The postings on www.Divorcenet.com express this clearly. One posting from "still searching" expresses the emotional trauma of a woman in her forties whose paternity is still not clear. Her mother had several affairs, so the daughter has had "a life of uncertainty" that has affected her marriage, her parenting skills, her job, and her emotional well-being.

Curiosity and Celebrity Testing

When DNA identity tests revealed the liaison between Thomas Jefferson and one of his slaves, Sally Hemings, this was "breaking news," although Jefferson scholars had long been aware of it. The case, widely reported in the media, became a huge political metaphor, a way to comment more generally on presidential indiscretions. It also provoked a moral debate about Jefferson's personal character and moral standing. Was he "the original deadbeat dad"? A ravenous press disrupted the private lives of family members, but it is only one of many cases in which human DNA remains—sometimes hair, sometimes body tissue—are tested to resolve historical mysteries, to rewrite history, and to support political or commercial agendas (Andrews and Nelkin 2001).

Many celebrities have been disinterred for DNA and other testing. Included are Zachary Taylor, Butch Cassidy, Francisco Pizarro, Napoleon, Lizzie Borden, Jesse James, Josef Mengele, and the last czar of Russia and his family. Even Tutankhamen (King Tut) got a paternity test in an effort to solve the mystery of who fathered the boy. Some of this postmortem testing of celebrities is simply to verify who is actually buried in a particular grave. Sometimes exhumation has revealed not only the identity of the body but also the cause of death. The exhumation and testing of celebrity bodies become media events, in effect, a forensic version of tabloid history, satisfying personal curiosity and meeting the cravings of celebrity watchers.

For some celebrity watchers, a curious case involved the story of a Thai monk accused of fathering the child of a follower. The woman sued him for paternity of the ten-year-old child, and the Buddhist council recommended the monk take a DNA test to clear up the scandal. The rumors, claimed Thai newspapers, were damaging the image of Buddhism, because monks must take a vow of celibacy. The monk, however, refused to take a paternity test (*New Straits Times* 1995).

Peace of Mind or Pandora's Box?

On November 6, 2000, the ABC show *20/20* featured Ben Gellar and his seven-year-old son, Bryan. Ben Gellar was married for twenty-one years and had two children in college when his wife became pregnant. But only four months after giving birth to Bryan, his wife died, and Ben became both father and mother to the child. Two years later, a stranger appeared at his home, claiming that he was Bryan's biological dad and demanding DNA paternity tests. He proved his biological relationship to the child and sued for custody. Rather than face a trial, Ben agreed to share custody, but he also had to pay child support. Meanwhile, Bryan, often against his will and too young to understand what had happened, began spending his weekends with a new family (Gellar 2000).

Through such stories, some media suggest that the revelations of paternity tests may open a Pandora's box. Does biological truth cause greater damage than deception? "It can break hearts." Occasionally critics are quoted. Joan Entmacher of the National Women's Law Center warns that "children will also be hurt when genetic tests disprove something that is the cornerstone of their identity" (quoted in Kaminer 2000, 63). Truth, writes a reporter, can be "an atom bomb" in a family (*St. Louis Post-Dispatch* 2000). But some observers have suggested that the practice might also constrain "studs" (Hax 2000).

Moreover, the information from the underwear, swabs, and other samples can be abused, for they can also be a source of information beyond identification. Samples, for example, can be tested to detect a person's health status or predisposition to genetic disease, exposing that person to genetic discrimination. Indeed, paternity testing, like the wider practice of storing DNA and tissue samples, is hardly benign.

The medias' enthusiasm and support for paternity testing masks many questions. What is a "real" parental relationship? What is the real importance of biological truth? Are there cases where it is better not to know? Does a society that encourages DNA testing really value its children? Or are children becoming pawns in parental disputes? Will divorces become more contentious and family ties more strained as media warnings arouse suspicion?

From the media reports and company ads, people expect biological testing to become a technological fix for family problems—a solution that will promote peace of mind. The tests are also touted as instruments that should be used in the courts. But should the best interests of the child, a basic assumption in family law, be trumped by biological evidence? How can the courts balance the rights of the man and the well-being of the child? Faced with many custody disputes, various courts have come out with different decisions concerning the relative importance of biological relationships. Will judges, pressed for time and responsive to popular opinion as well as to scientific consensus, accept genetic evidence as the bottom line? Media commentaries suggest again and again that the law has not kept up with the realities of science (Lewin 2001). But should it? Is not parenthood more than DNA? If you care for a child for years should you have to "de-bond?"

My files are now swamped with media stories, company ads, and news reports, and my computer is bookmarked with many Web sites—most rather hysterical, some rather bemused. But, I wonder, what in fact is the issue? Has family life ever been neat and tidy? Have not purse strings and heartstrings always been at stake in the dynamics of both troubled and "normal" families? What, after all, is so new and so newsworthy about paternity tests—except for the dominance of marketing media and the growing practice of consumer manipulation?

ACKNOWLEDGMENTS

Thanks to Leah Belsky and Mary Anderlik Majumder for providing many of the examples on which this chapter is based.

BIBLIOGRAPHY

Andrews, L., and D. Nelkin. 2001. *Body Bazaar: The Market for Human Tissue in the Biotechnology Age.* New York: Crown Publishers.

Associated Press. 1997. DNA labs offer new test of family ties. *Augusta Chronicle,* 19 March (online).

Barash, D., and J. Lipton. 2001. *The Myth of Monogamy: Fidelity and Infidelity in Animals and People.* New York: W. H. Freeman.

Belluck, P. 1997. Paternity testing for fun and profit. *New York Times,* 3 August.

Birkhead, T. 2000. *Promiscuity.* Cambridge: Harvard University Press.

Citizens against Paternity Fraud. 2001. www.PaternityFraud.com.

Ferguson, C. 2001. DNA testing can be a dirty job. *Tennessean,* 15 April.

Finkler, K. 2001. The kin in the gene: The medicalization of the family and kinship in American society. *Current Anthropology* 42:235–63.

Fulghum, R. 1995. Going home again. *Sky,* May.

Gellar, B. 2000. Interview. *Chicago Sun Times,* 5 September.

Goodman, E. 2001. What makes a father? *Boston Globe,* 4 May.

Goodman, W. 1990. Giving up a child: Being given up. *New York Times,* 28 November.

Gumbel, B. 2001. *The Early Show.* CBS, 18 April (transcript).

Hax, C. 2000. Tell me about it. *Washington Post,* 25 June.

Identigene. 2005. www.identigene.com/SWIMX.

Kaminer, W. 2000. Fathers in court. *American Prospect* 11(21):62–63.

Kaye, K. 1980. Turning two identities into one. *Psychology Today,* November, 46–50.

Kelleher, K. 2001. Paternity testing is not about genetics but about trust and fairness. *Los Angeles Times,* 9 April.

Landers, A. 2000. DNA test could answer paternity question. *San Francisco Chronicle,* 5 December.

Lewin, T. 2001. In genetic testing for paternity, law often lags behind science. *New York Times,* 11 March.

Mirabella, L. 1997. Lab's tests give answers to genetic questions. *Baltimore Sun,* 25 November.

Montel Williams Show. 1997. New York, 6 November.

Nelkin, D. 1994. *Selling Science: How the Press Covers Science and Technology,* 2nd ed. New York: W. H. Freeman.

Nelkin, D., and S. Lindee. 1995. *The DNA Mystique: The Gene as Cultural Icon.* New York: W. H. Freeman.

New Straits Times. 1995. Thai monk refuses DNA test. 7 February.

Norton, C. 2000. Faceless fathers may be identified. *Independent News,* 24 April.

Rogers, L. 2000. Who's your daddy? *Ottawa Citizen,* 21 June.

Schneider, D. 1968. *American Kinship.* Englewood Cliffs, NJ: Prentice Hall.

Smith, C. 2001. Stop paternity fraud petition. www.Petitiononline.com.

Spector, H. 1999. Ad for paternity testing raises eyebrows. *New Orleans Times-Picayune,* 8 August.

St. Louis Post-Dispatch. 2000. DNA should determine support. 20 May.

Starnes, R. 1998. Latest weapon in legal arsenal is all in the genes. *Ottawa Citizen,* 13 March.

Taylor, J. 2000. Feminism—will men be able to sue? *Sunday Times* (London), 11 June. www.mail-archive.com/CTRL@listserv.aol.com/msg45082.html.

Tiger, L. 1999. *The Decline of Males.* New York: Golden Books.

Wade, N. 2001. Birds do it. Bees do it. Some people do too. *New York Times,* 21 May.

Weizel, R. 1991. First person: A voice from the past. *Parenting,* October, 90.

Zoglin, R., and C. Faltermayer. 1997. From here to paternity. *Time,* 11 August.

CHAPTER TWO

Three Meanings of Parenthood

Thomas H. Murray, Ph.D.

Here is a very sad story. A man and woman seek and are granted a divorce, with all its customary grief over the division of property, support, and other financial tussles. Two years later the man has himself and his four-year-old son subjected to genetic relationship testing and learns that his son is not his biological child. A few months later the man informs the boy that he is not his biological offspring and cuts off his relationship with the boy (Dolgin 2000).

In another case, a man discovers that three of the four children born during his marriage, which ended three years previously, are not his biological offspring. He won custody of all four children during the divorce and cared for them until giving over custody to his former wife when, he says, his travel schedule overwhelmed him. Soon after, he underwent a test to determine whether he is a carrier of cystic fibrosis, a disease his youngest son has inherited. The test shows the man is not a carrier. He asks to be freed from paying child support. The judge, in a strange ruling, compels him to continue to supply child support but cuts off his visitation rights. The man's attorney draws this lesson: "I now advise every man who's getting a divorce to get paternity testing. I don't like it much, but now it seems like it could be malpractice not to warn them" (Lewin 2001).

There are layers of sadness in these stories. Divorces themselves are occasions for sadness, especially when children are involved. The children's losses are doubled. Not only are their parents divorcing, but the men they have known their entire lives as their fathers have, in the first case, renounced them and, in the second, been cut off by the order of a judge. We must add one more terrible sadness to this list: the man—once husband to the woman, father to the children—is deprived of his relationship to those children. That man's loss, I believe, is as great as the children's.

I know very little about the character of these particular father-child relationships. But I do know this: if a man and a child have lived together, have believed each other to be father and son or daughter, then whatever relationship they have had, however loving or distant, warm or contentious, is profoundly important to them both. For that is the nature of what it is to live as parent and child.

In these sad stories, two meanings of parenthood—genetic and rearing—are discovered to diverge. This happens often enough. There are no reliable measures for the incidence of what is called, blandly, "misattributed paternity." Such a passionless label bleaches out the background of desire, deception, and betrayal that often lies behind the pale facts and that inspires agony columns, bathetic talk shows, the "duped dads" movement, and, occasionally, great art. For the United States, estimates of misattributed paternity range from less than 5 percent to more than 10 percent of all children. Less well known is the phenomenon of misattributed *maternity*. It is likely very rare, but it does happen. I've made it a practice, over the years, of asking clinical geneticists whether they have seen any cases of misattributed maternity; every genetics department seems to have had such a case.

Given the proliferation of assisted reproductive technologies and other reproductive arrangements, such as commercial surrogacy, it is wise to add a third meaning of parenthood—intention—to the more familiar pair of genetic and rearing (or social) parenthood. In what follows I attempt to sort out these three meanings of parenthood, reflect on the moral grounding that might be given to each of them, and consider how each stands up against the three models of the parent-child relationship that I proposed in *The Worth of a Child:* the child as property, the parent as steward, and parent-child mutuality (Murray 1996).

Parenthood as Genetics

Biology—or, more colloquially, blood—has long been accorded great significance as the source of the fundamental tie between parent and child (Grossberg 2001). We think we know what we mean by identifying someone as a genetic parent, but digging deeper into the notion turns up complexities. A genetic parent contributes half of a child's DNA, right? Of course, there is the matter of mitochondrial DNA—more on that shortly; and there is less DNA in the father's Y chromosome than in either parent's X chromosome, so if the child is male, less than half of his total DNA comes from the father. So let us hedge somewhat: the genetic parent contributes more or less half of the child's DNA. Each biological grandparent, meanwhile, has contributed a quarter, on average, of the child's DNA. Does that make them half genetic parents? No, we say. It must be a direct and immediate contribution, not mediated through one's descendants.

But there are new techniques that complicate matters. Ooplasm transplant involves taking a bit of cytoplasm from an egg of a relatively young, healthy woman and injecting it into an egg of a woman who has had difficulty conceiving. In the cytoplasmic soup are many mitochondria, the energy factories of the cell, each carrying its own tiny genome. Is the woman from whose egg the mitochondria were sucked out a third genetic parent of the child conceived from the egg with the donated cytoplasm? If the criterion is a direct and immediate contribution of DNA or genes, the answer must be yes.

Pending further developments, we seem to have four ways to be a biological parent, of which three count as "genetic"—providing egg, sperm, or mitochondria are the genetic means; providing a womb is surely biological, but not in itself genetic. So, gestation is biological but not genetic; providing the egg is genetic and usually, but not always, linked to gestation; and sperm are genetic and never—at least not yet—derived from the same individual who provides a womb.

Reproductive cloning would provide yet another way to be a genetic parent. In reproductive cloning one person provides the nuclear DNA and another person supplies the enucleated egg. There are many reasons to doubt the practical feasibility and ethical justifiability of human reproductive cloning. Even if it were possible to do successful reproductive cloning, it would change nothing in this analysis. Instances of reproductive cloning would require a sorting out of biology, intention, and rearing, just as in other cases in which children are conceived and adults navigate the details of parenthood.

There are two meanings of parenthood in addition to the biological. Parenthood as *intention,* with or without biology, with or without rearing the child, is not a new concept, but it has become vastly more common with the proliferation of assisted reproductive technologies and vastly more influential as concepts such as procreative liberty have become popular frameworks for thinking about the law and ethics of reproductive technologies.

For the idea of parenthood grounded in caring for the child and the relationship that grows from such caring, consider the well-known children's story *The Velveteen Rabbit*. The rabbit of the title is made from cloth and stuffing. The child loves the Velveteen Rabbit, which becomes his constant companion. In time, the power of that love, tested by illness and separation, transforms the inanimate stuffed animal into a real rabbit. Does the love between an adult—who may or may not have any biological tie—and a child create, in time, a "real" parent?

Parenthood as Intention

Many sorts of intentions may result in the creation of a child; these intentions can intersect with biology and with rearing, but they can exist independent of either or both. An adult can, for example, intend to bring a child into the world with no commitment to having anything to do with caring for that child. The intention may be linked thus to biology with no connection to rearing. Or the intent could be to bring a child into the world with no direct biological connection but with a wholehearted commitment to raising that child. In artificial insemination by donor the would-be rearing father has no biological link to his offspring. In egg donation with the male partner's sperm in in vitro fertilization, the would-be rearing mother has no genetic connection to the child. If she is the gestational mother, then she has that as a biological relationship, but if a gestational surrogate is employed (I mean that in its commercial as well as its generic sense) and the process does not use the would-be rearing mother's egg, then no biological tie exists.

In practice, much of the appeal of the infertility industry to couples intending to have a child is the prospect of creating one with a genetic tie to one or both of the adults. Other constellations of intentions and possibilities arise as well. It is possible to sponsor the creation of a child with no biological tie to either putative parent. The couple may have a variety of intentions: to avoid an inheritable disease carried by one or both adults; to get around the difficulties often encountered in adoption, especially adoptions of healthy infants; to be able to choose genetic parents that have characteristics desirable in the eyes of the would-be rearing parents.

I hesitate to describe this next scenario. An individual or a couple selects the gamete providers, secures gestational services, and then arranges for the resulting child to be raised by yet other adults. Why do I hesitate? Because a quarter-century of working in bioethics has taught me to beware of absurd, far-fetched hypothetical cases—they often turn out to be true. I don't know of such a case. But the profit-oriented, whatever-the-client-desires ethos of many IVF centers makes me wonder what would happen if someone made such a request—and was willing to pay for it.

People's intentions to become a parent may have nothing to do with the child's creation. Adopting an already-born child presupposes nothing about biological ties between the child and the adults who become its parents. We need to exercise care in how we describe the likely absence of biological relationship in adoption. I have heard accounts, difficult to verify but plausible in the light of the complexity of human relationships and actions, of a couple adopting a child who may be the man's biological offspring. It is easy to imagine the seething brew of ambivalence, resentment, anger, betrayal, and revenge that such an arrangement might create. But whatever its potential complexities, adoption also shows that rearing parenthood can exist independent of either biology or any intention to create a child.

Parenthood as Rearing Relationship

Genetic or other biological connection is neither necessary nor sufficient to make a parent-child relationship. In adoption, formal or informal, the relevant intention is to become a parent, not to create a child. The intention is to initiate a relationship. There are three key features of the idea of parenthood as a rearing relationship.

1. *There must be an appropriate acknowledgment of the relationship.* In ancient Rome, the practice of taking children into one's household could result in their being embraced as *alumni* or *alumnae*. In the United States, formal legal adoption was uncommon until the mid nineteenth century, because the laws of the various states did not provide for it; a special act of the legislature was required for legal recognition of such parent-child relationships (Grossberg 1985). For children born to a couple recognized as married, the child is presumed to be the issue of the marriage, and the rights and responsibilities of parenthood are ascribed to the couple.

2. *There is a powerful emotional connection between the rearing adult and the child.* This connection is typically intense and lifelong. It is complex and, at times, one sided. Parents can be attentive and devoted or hopelessly self-centered. Most parents are some mixture of loving devotion and narcissistic self-absorption. Children may take their parents for granted or treat them

with loving considerateness. We should neither denigrate nor idealize the emotional bonds between parents and children. The point here is that these bonds, in all their complexity and occasional ambivalence, are vitally important in the lives of parents and children. Indeed, the failure to establish or sustain such connections is likely to be a painful and fundamental deficit in our lives.

3. *The rearing parents must engage in those practices of caring judged appropriate in that time and place.* Here I mean caring in its broadest sense of providing for all or for a significant portion of the needs of the developing child, from basic support and physical care to nourishing the child's emotional and intellectual development and ensuring that the child acquires the skills needed for independent living.

All three threads—biological, intentional, and rearing—can be woven together tightly in a parent-child relationship. Nonetheless, they are distinguishable in practice as well as in principle and have been so for millennia. The methods for separating biology from intention and rearing have multiplied, and the legal provisions for recognizing rearing relationships in the absence of biological ones have been made routine. Reflecting on the new choices being forced upon us by a combination of the technology of genetic relationship testing and laws made in earlier eras, we may find it helpful to consider the possible moral groundings for each of these meanings.

Possible Moral Groundings for Three Meanings of Parenthood

Genetic Parenthood

One possible strategy for portraying genetic parenthood as a morally defensible concept is to claim that there is a property right to a child vested in the genetic progenitor. The ancient Roman idea of *patria potestas* asserted a broad right over persons and property—including children—held by the eldest male in the family (Grossberg 1985). Note that this is not identical to the idea that the child's immediate biological parents held such a right. For one thing, only males held this power. For another, control was in the hands of the oldest living male progenitor, who could be the grandfather or even the great-grandfather (although, given the brief life expectancies for men of that era, the fathers were far more likely to be alive than their predecessors). Abandoned children were *res vacantes,* unclaimed objects, in Roman law. Roman fathers retained rights over even their abandoned biological offspring until 331 A.D., when Constantine ruled that such children were under the authority of their rearing parents. The moral claim, then, resides in some version of the argument that children are property, their genetic progenitors are the proper owners, and therefore the owners have a powerful first claim over their child/property.

Ethically speaking, a defense of the primacy of genetic parenthood by invoking the idea of the child as the property of its genetic parents is a nonstarter. Any contemporary account of morality that failed to acknowledge that children were *not* property and that children's interests and well-being mattered would be found grievously defective. The few theorists who argue for a less-than-full status for children—usually for a very brief interval after birth—bear a heavy burden of persuasion. This is so because the independent moral significance of children, even newborn infants, is such a broadly shared and fundamental tenet of morality. If children were property, they would not have such moral standing. Interestingly, the Roman concept of *patria potestas* included the discretion to kill one's children, yet this act seems to have been regarded with great moral disapproval. Even in the heyday of *patria potestas,* then, the child was not reduced to mere property, disposable at the whim of its owner.

Our laws lag well behind our ethics on this score. I will have more to say about the stories of Baby Jessica and Baby Richard, because they illuminate the persistent strength of a father's power over his offspring. Both children were surrendered for adoption by their biological mothers. In both cases the man whom genetic testing showed to be the biological father asserted his claim to the child, despite the child having spent the first years of his or her life knowing only the would-be adoptive couple as its parents. And in both cases the genetic fathers were able to gain custody of children who, whatever their biological ties, were strangers to them, because the men had never legally surrendered their paternal rights—and because American family law privileged biological relationships over years-long relationships of caring and nurturing.

As I write this, my granddaughter Grace Emilia is two-and-a-half, roughly the age of Jessica and Richard when the courts ordered them to be removed from their rearing parents and turned over to their biological fathers. Grace is being raised by her biological parents. But I doubt that this fact of biology makes any discernible difference in Grace's profound attachment to her mother and father. I can scarcely imagine the pain that would be caused if Grace were taken from her parents and given to someone else to be raised—pain to Grace, but, as important, pain to the mother and father who love her. Why should we believe that the pain experienced by Jessica and her rearing parents, or by Richard and his rearing parents, was notably less? Reforms of U.S. adoption law are in process, as is a reevaluation of the marital presumption of paternity (Glennon 2000).

Another possible line of argument for parenthood as biology is what we might call *naturalistic prerational explanations.* A prime example of such an argument is a variation of the "selfish gene" idea: that, somehow, being raised by one's genetic parents is an expression of a pervasive and powerful natural force and may be highly advantageous to the child. The advantage comes from being raised by adults with a strong disposition to care for the child, that disposition deriving its potency from natural selection as a means of assuring that the parents' genes survive. This is not, to be sure, a moral argument. It could be incorporated into a more complex argument such as this: (1) the survival of children is a good consequence, (2) factors favoring that survival should be given precedence, (3) (factual premise) genetic ties between rearing parents and children favor child survival notably more successfully than do ties between rearing though nongenetic parents and their children, and therefore (4) genetic ties should be given precedence.

Skolnick (1998) describes the pervasiveness of such latent assumptions in American law and their dangers: "Many commentators . . . believe that the child's best interests are in fact served by growing up with biological parents, and that parents not only have a right to their children but that 'natural bonds of affection' lead parents to care for their children in a way that no 'stranger' could. This biological slant of the legal system also reflects widespread, but usually unarticulated assumptions about ties based on blood and genes in American culture. Because they are so taken for granted, there is a danger that unless they are made explicit, these assumptions may well guide decision making and discussion of the issues in an unreflective way" (238–39). For this argument to be persuasive there would have to be good evidence (not mere assertion) that the factual premise is true. We would also have to weigh the dubious claims about enhanced child survival against other goods that we seek and interests that deserve moral and legal protection.

Another version of this sort of argument is that children benefit when they resemble their parents. This is in part tied to the stigma attached to adoption or any other nonbiological parent-child relationship (Bartholet 1999). But, of course, as the stigma eases there is less to worry about when children do not look just like their parents. More commonly, it is assumed that the benefit comes from the parent's narcissistic investment in the child. The parent presumably sees herself or himself reflected in the child's eyes, face, or demeanor. This assertion is, I believe, at best incomplete. I cannot speak for all parents, but I suspect that we spend much more time looking at our spouses than at ourselves. In that sense, what we may see reflected in our children is the image of our partner, not so much our self-portrait. As a convincing moral argument, in any event, this one has the same weaknesses as the selfish-gene claim.

Parenthood as Intention

The intention to have and raise a child as a manifestation of autonomous choice has a powerful ideological resonance in contemporary American culture. Just as the autonomy of patients became the rallying cry and first-among-equals moral principle in the early years of the modern medical ethics movement, so a variant of autonomy dubbed "procreative liberty" has served as a justification for practices in the infertility industry (Robertson 1994). (Procreative liberty's adequacy as a moral framework for comprehending all that is ethically significant in reproductive technology and practices has come under attack, as has autonomy's primacy in understanding a host of issues in bioethics [Annas 1998; Murray 2002].) The key to parenthood as intention is the uncoerced, informed, and voluntary choice of the adult or adults who, for whatever reasons, decide to have a child.

Parenthood as intention is a clear component of adoption. Adoption is the intentional creation of a parent-child relationship without regard to biological ties. Things become murkier in the much more commonplace cases of parent-child relationships created the old-fashioned way. Although many children are, as the saying goes, wanted children, not all are. Some children enter the world because their biological parents did nothing to prevent them from doing so. The parents may be pleased, ambivalent, or distraught. Some children are conceived as a consequence of failed contraception; their subsequent birth may or may not be the result of a conscious choice not to abort, but it would be misleading to say that this was parenthood by intention. In fact, the intention was at least initially the opposite—to avoid having a child.

In the end, a great many parent-child relationships have a strong component of intention in their makeup. But not all, and not always unambiguously. Many children are conceived not because there was an intention to have a child but as an unintended consequence of sexual intercourse. A foreseeable consequence for the most part. But foreseeability is not the same thing as intention. Whatever one's views about the desirability of making every child an expressly wanted—that is, intended—child, there is no good reason to believe that parent-child relationships created through inadvertence are for that reason morally inferior to those created through careful intention.

Parenthood as intention, then, may be a desirable practice if it results in happier, healthier, and more vital children along with committed, loving, thriving parents. But it is not a necessary condition for establishing a parent-child relationship, nor does intention inevitably distinguish good relationships from bad ones. People who intend the birth of a child may be wonderful parents or indifferent or even horrible ones. People who become parents without specifically intending to do so can likewise be indifferent or bad parents, or they can discover deep wellsprings of love and patience. That a person intended to become a parent of this child may provide additional moral grounds for holding her or him accountable and responsible for the child, but it does not clearly entitle that person to specific rights to the child greater than the rights of a parent by inadvertence who nevertheless becomes a devoted rearing parent. Nor does the absence of intention in itself diminish either parental responsibilities or parental rights.

Parenthood as Rearing

Humans are born into a state of total dependency on those who care for them. Children remain mostly dependent for many years. For most adults, the response to a child's dependency is natural and unforced. This is not to say that caring for an infant is easy or that parents never know exhaustion, frustration, and resentment at the burdens of infant and child care. The amazing thing is how, in the face of these burdens and frustrations, adults come to love and cherish their children. An adult stranger who entered one's life making similar demands on one's time, energy, and attention might be resented and tossed out. But children, in their dependency, evoke love and caring.

This is assuredly part of our evolutionary heritage. The intensity and near universality of parental love is not a recent cultural creation. The late historian John Boswell, in his history of child abandonment (1988), wrote, "Everywhere in Western culture, from religious literature to secular poetry, parental love is invoked as the ultimate standard of selfless and untiring devotion, central metaphors of theology and ethics presuppose this love as a universal point of reference, and language must devise special terms to characterize persons wanting in this 'natural' affection" (37–38).

What makes this an ethical point rather than a biological observation or historical curiosity is the role of such caring relationships in human flourishing. From the child's point of view, failing to receive consistent, devoted care is devastating and potentially lethal. For children who survive despite indifferent parenting, life is immensely more difficult than it needs to be. Children's future possibilities for flourishing are impaired when they are not loved, guided, and prepared for adult life. A great many adults (some might say all emotionally healthy adults) in turn experience enduring relationships that embody deep commitments and wide-ranging mutual obligations as central and essential parts of their own flourishing. Rearing and loving children is perhaps the most common but by no means the only way of creating those relationships.

Human flourishing, an important moral concept at least since Aristotle, is deeply intertwined with parenting as rearing and caring. This is true not only for the children whose capacities for flourishing are shaped by the care they receive but also for the adults who provide the care. Genetic parenthood's ties to flourishing are distant and dim. However selfish our genes may be, the mere fact that some of one's genes are surviving seems to have little or no connection to one's flourishing. Imagine two men. The first man conceived a child with a woman in a brief affair and by mutual agreement has had nothing to do with either the child or its mother for the child's entire life. The second man and his wife raised from infancy an adopted child whom they love very much. What if, tragically, these children died? Whose lives are devastated? Or change the story slightly so that the second man married the first child's mother and raised the child as his own. At the child's death, it is the rearing parents who have suffered the life-altering loss. The genetic father may feel something, but in the absence of any relationship with the child it will be of an entirely different and lesser order.

The connection of parenthood as intention to flourishing flows directly from parenthood as rearing. Even the advocates of procreative liberty frame their case in terms of creating a child *for the purpose of raising* the child. The desire to have a biological link to the child is in the service of the anticipated rearing relationship, not an end in itself. The test case would be the hypothetical case described earlier: when a couple wants their gametes used to create a child so that their genes live on, but with no intention of raising the child.

A crucial point here should not be lost: raising, caring for, and loving a child contributes as much to the adults' flourishing as it does to the child's. Would-be parents therefore have profoundly important moral interests in being rearing parents. Adults may have legitimate interests in genetic parenthood and in parenthood as intention also. But note the change in moral tone when we move to rearing parenthood. The focus is not on the adult's rights or autonomous choices but on the place of enduring and indeed demanding relationships of caring in the flourishing of adults. I noted in *The Worth of a Child* the irony of trying to understand what is morally important about parenthood through the prism of autonomy. Becoming a caring and engaged parent means freely choosing (for those who enter parenthood freely) a life with deeply constrained freedom. Marriage can change one's life; having children alters it radically and irrevocably.

Parenthood as engagement in caring for a child fits our experience better than does genetic parenting or parenting as intention. It acknowledges and embraces the significance of enduring commitments and relationships in human flourishing—an honorable and important concept in ethics. And it recognizes the importance to children of reliable bonds to caring adults.

Three Models of the Parent-Child Relationship

In *The Worth of a Child,* I proposed three models of the relationship between parent and child: the child as property, the parent as steward, and parent-child mutuality. How do the three meanings of parenthood stack up against these models of the parent-child relationship?

The Child as Property

We no longer accept the near-absolute power over one's offspring conferred by the ancient Romans under *patria potestas*. Roman law did not have the same direct impact on the development of the common law traditions shared by Britain and the United States as it had on other Western legal systems. But the notion of the parent's—or more precisely, the father's—rights over his offspring echoes the Roman privilege accorded the patriarch. According to Michael Grossberg's *Governing the Hearth* (1985), the English common law tradition inherited by the United States regarded children as "assets of paternal estates in which fathers had vested interests. As dependent, subordinate beings, their services, earnings, and the like became the property of their paternal masters in exchange for life and maintenance" (25).

In chapter 7 of this volume, Grossberg describes the complex evolution of American family law and the concepts and standards devised by the law to assign the rights and responsibilities of parenthood. Until the advent of scientific tests—highly imprecise at first, now remarkably accurate with DNA relationship testing—courts had few reliable methods to ascertain biological fatherhood. The "four seas" rule or other proof that a husband had no access to his wife was about as definitive as one could get. The marital presumption—that any issue of a married woman was the child of her husband—held dominion (Glennon 2000). The property-like rights as well as the responsibilities of fatherhood flowed from a social arrangement—marriage. From the state's perspective, the marital presumption solved many problems. That the marital presumption was rebuttable—however difficult rebuttal might be—implies that biological fatherhood was the underlying principle. DNA testing offers near-certain evidence of genetic parenthood, and so the marital presumption has gone from being solid to wobbly to scientifically (at least) irrelevant. If we continue to assign parental rights and responsibilities according to a social status such as marriage, it will be for ethical and social policy reasons, not because marriage is the most reliable marker of genetic parentage.

Until recently, American adoption law reflected the idea that the child is property of its genetic parents. Baby Jessica and Baby Richard were both taken from their rearing parents and handed over to their genetic fathers because neither man had formally relinquished his legal rights to have custody of his offspring, despite the absence of intention or any rearing relationship. To the courts, unrelinquished genetic fatherhood was sufficient reason to overturn a completed adoption in Baby Richard's case. Baby Jessica's formal adoption was in process when her genetic father intervened, and it was never completed. On 30 July 1993 the U.S. Supreme Court ruled against the DeBoers, who had cared for Jessica since birth. Justice John Paul Stevens wrote for the majority that "the Iowa courts determined that the parental rights of the child's biological father had not been terminated . . . and that therefore applicants were not entitled to adopt the child" (*DeBoer v. DeBoer* 1993). Justice Harry Blackmun, joined by Justice Sandra Day O'Connor, wrote in dissent,

"This is a case that touches the raw nerves of life's relationships. We have before us, in Jessica, a child of tender years who for her entire life has been nurtured by the DeBoers, a loving couple led to believe through the adoption process and the then-single-mother's consent, that Jessica was theirs. Now, the biological father appears, marries the mother, and claims paternal status towards Jessica." Acknowledging his uncertainty, Justice Blackmun nonetheless wrote that he was "not willing to wash my hands of this case at this stage, with the personal vulnerability of the child so much at risk."

Parenthood as genetic is aligned closely with the idea of the child as property. Parenthood as intention fits less well, although some practices by the infertility industry steer worrisomely close. The more the child is treated as a commodity, the more parenthood resembles the child-as-property model of parent-child relationships. Rearing parenthood, in contrast, leaves the child-as-property model far behind.

The Parent as Steward

According to the Oxford English Dictionary, a steward is "an official who controls the domestic affairs of a household, supervising the service of his master's table, directing the domestics, and regulating houseful expenditure." The parent-as-steward looks morally more palatable than the child-as-property model. It limits sharply what the parent can do to the child—no selling into slavery, for one thing. But it leaves open the question, for whom is the steward managing the child: for God, the state, the child herself or himself? But the most significant shortcoming of the parent-as-steward model is its failure to capture adequately what is at the heart of the parent-child bond. A good steward, after all, needs to be disinterested—that is, the steward should be pursuing the master's interests, not his or her own. Nor do we worry much about the welfare, interests, or flourishing of the steward. When it comes to parents and children, though, we prize the deep emotional intimacy of their relationships and their mutual flourishing, not the child's well-being in isolation.

For all its limitations, how does the parent-as-steward model match up with parenthood as genetic, as intention, or as rearing? Genetics, or biology more broadly, hinges on the origin of the ties, not on the norms or practices governing the ongoing relationship, so whether the parent has a genetic tie to the child has no direct relevance to the parent-as-steward model. Intention can merely describe the origins of the relationship, but here we can state again a distinction between two broad sorts of intentions. First would be the intention to create a child (with or without specific genetic ties to the intending parents). Second would be the intention to incorporate that child into one's life—to raise that child. Intentions of the first type, in the absence of intentions to raise the child, seem bizarre and worthy of neither moral respect nor legal protection. The parent-as-steward captures in part the second sort of intention at its best—the commitment to the child's well-being and ultimate flourishing. In that sense it resembles rearing parenthood. The problem with the stewardship model is its incompleteness, its indifference to the flourishing of the steward and to the centrality of the relationship of the caretaker to the cared-for child.

Parent-Child Mutuality

Regarding parents and children through the prism of mutuality cuts through simplistic assumptions about human motivation and penetrates to the core of what people experience in healthy parent-child relationships. When I aim at my child's well-being there is no denying that I benefit in two ways: my child's flourishing gives me joy, and I become a more capable, mature, compassionate, and insightful person. It only works when my principal motive is to help my child; yet I know that in doing so I advance my own flourishing as well. The concept, borrowed from Erik Erikson, is *mutuality* (Erikson 1964).

Mutuality is true to the emotional and psychological nature of the parent-child relationship. It is compatible with human flourishing as a moral goal. Indeed, if it is true for most or all of us that our flourishing requires enduring, loving relationships, then raising children in a loving manner is crucial both to their flourishing and to ours. How, then, does mutuality relate to the three meanings of parenthood?

Genetic parenthood is incidental to parent-child mutuality. To the extent that a genetic tie enhances the growth of mutuality and the flourishing of parents and children, it deserves to be valued. But it is neither necessary nor sufficient. Parenthood as intention is related to parent-child mutuality in a similar way. Like genetic parenthood, to the extent that intention facilitates mutuality it is a good thing. In the treatment of infertility, where parenthood as intention is the norm, would-be parents are presumably seeking to have children because they understand in some fashion that their own flourishing is enhanced by having and raising a child.

The key to parenthood as mutuality is caring for, raising, and loving a child—what I have called "rearing parenthood." Because parent-child mutuality is the model that best captures what is morally central in parenthood, and because mutual flourishing is the appropriate ethical standard, then rearing parenthood is the meaning of parenthood we should honor most highly in our customs and protect most fiercely in our laws.

BIBLIOGRAPHY

Annas, G. 1998. Human cloning: A choice or an echo? *University of Dayton Law Review* 23:247–75.

Bartholet, E. 1999. *Family Bonds: Adoption, Infertility, and the New World of Child Production*. Boston: Beacon Press.

Boswell, J. 1988. *The Kindness of Strangers: The Abandonment of Children in Western Europe from Late Antiquity to the Renaissance*. New York: Pantheon Press.

DeBoer v. DeBoer. 1993. 509 U.S. 1301.

Dolgin, J. L. 2000. Choice, tradition, and the new genetics: The fragmentation of the ideology of family. *Connecticut Law Review* 32:523–66.

Erikson, E. H. 1964. Human strength and the cycle of generations. In *Insight and Responsibility*, 109–157. New York: Norton.

Glennon, T. 2000. Somebody's child: Evaluating the erosion of the marital presumption of paternity. *West Virginia Law Review* 102:555–59.

Grossberg, M. 1985. *Governing the Hearth: Law and Family in Nineteenth Century America*. Chapel Hill: University of North Carolina Press.

———. 2001. How to give the present a past? Family law in the United States 1950–2000. In *Cross Currents: Family Law and Policy in the United States and England*, ed. M. Maclean, 3–29. Oxford: Oxford University Press.

Lewin, T. 2001. In genetic testing for paternity, law often lags behind science. *New York Times*, 11 March.

Murray, T. H. 1996. *The Worth of a Child*. Berkeley and Los Angeles: University of California Press.

———. 2002. What are families for? Getting to an ethics of reproductive technologies. *Hastings Center Report* 32(3):41–45.

Robertson, J. A. 1994. *Children of Choice: Freedom and the New Reproductive Technologies*. Princeton: Princeton University Press.

Skolnick, A. 1998. Solomon's children: The new biologism, psychological parenthood, attachment theory, and the best interest standard. In *All Our Families: New Policies for a New Century: A Report of the Berkeley Family Forum*, ed. S. D. Sugarman, 236–255. Oxford: Oxford University Press.

CHAPTER THREE

Ethical Issues in DNA-Based Paternity Testing

Jeffrey Blustein, Ph.D.

The Uses of DNA Paternity Testing: Some Scenarios

Sometimes, a presumptive father's discovery that he is not biologically related to the child he has assumed is "his" occurs unexpectedly, as a result of carrier testing for a genetic disorder or testing for suitability as an organ donor. In other cases, determination of paternity (or nonpaternity) is the goal of testing, and with the advent of direct DNA testing, paternity can be established or disproved to an almost conclusive degree. DNA-based paternity testing is sought by presumptive as well as biological fathers, by men who are married or not married to the mother of the child, and by unmarried and married mothers. Consider the following scenarios, divided into four categories.

Category 1: Paternity testing with the aim of providing relief from parental obligations. In case I, Joe is married to Lynn and has developed a substantial parent-child relationship with her biological child. He seeks DNA paternity testing either before or during a divorce proceeding to relieve himself of post-divorce child support obligations. In one variant of this case (Ia), no biological father would be available to provide support should Joe's paternity be disproved; in a second variant (Ib), the biological father would be available. In case II, Carl is married to Eva, but has been an absent father and has no significant relationship with her biological child. He seeks DNA paternity testing under the same circumstances and for the same reason as in case I. There are also two variants of this case (IIa, IIb) that parallel those in case I.

Category 2: Paternity testing with the aim of imposing parental obligations. In case III, Bob and Francine have an on-again off-again relationship. Francine becomes pregnant, but Bob denies that he is the father and that he has any obligations to the child. He points out that he and Francine are not married and that he has never encouraged her to believe he has a long-term commitment to her. Francine wants a DNA test to force Bob to support the child.

Category 3: Paternity testing with the aim of denying parental rights. In case IV, Jim and Linda are getting a divorce. Linda seeks to contest her husband's paternity so that she can deny him the right to continue his relationship with her biological child.

Category 4: Paternity testing with the aim of asserting parental rights. In case V, George is not married to Jean, but he challenges the paternity of Jean's husband. He seeks DNA testing to establish his paternity and to assert his right to have a relationship with his biological child. In one variant of this case (Va), George seeks to establish and does establish his paternity shortly after the birth of the child; in another variant (Vb), George's paternity is established several years after the child's birth, during which time Jean's husband has formed a significant relationship with the child.

As these scenarios make clear, DNA paternity testing can be sought under a variety of circumstances and for various reasons. We can ask two questions at this point. (1) Are there good and sufficient reasons for restricting fathers' *access* to DNA-based paternity testing for the purpose of proving or disproving paternity? (2) Are there good and sufficient reasons for restricting the *use* of whatever information is or might be gained from DNA-based identity testing for the purpose of relieving/imposing parental obligations or asserting/denying parental rights? These are different questions that might have different answers, because one could argue both that fathers who want to know the truth about their paternity should be able to acquire this information *and* that, in some circumstances, evidence of paternity or nonpaternity should not be used (or admitted by a court of law) to absolve presumed fathers of parental obligations or to allow biological fathers to assert parental rights.

This chapter focuses on the uses of DNA-based paternity information and sets aside the question of a father's right to know the truth about his paternity. Even if there are sound moral reasons for restricting access to DNA testing, the reality is that it is becoming increasingly difficult to prevent individuals from acquiring this information. Access could be somewhat controlled were the law to permit DNA paternity testing only under a court order and only by a physician, and if there were penalties for physicians who did paternity testing without it. However, this is not the case at present. Increasingly, laboratories are marketing DNA paternity tests directly to the public and offering "curiosity testing," designed for private individuals who want DNA paternity information for their own purposes. Such testing is not done under a court order and is often conducted without any professional medical involvement.

The Significance of Biology for Determining Parental Obligations

To answer the question about the appropriate use of DNA-based paternity testing, one must consider the important but limited role of biological (and specifically genetic) relatedness in grounding parental obligations and rights. A common way of incurring parental obligations is to undertake them, and a standard way of undertaking parental obligations is to decide to procreate. In our society, decisions to procreate are not just decisions to produce a child, with no strings attached, but entail a commitment to rear the child or, if unwilling or unable to do so, to arrange for the child's upbringing by others. Merely playing a causal role in the creation of a child does not give rise to parental obligations, of course, for one can imagine circumstances in which an individual in no way consented to or had control over becoming a parent. (Consider the case of a woman who becomes pregnant as a result of rape and is forced to have the child.) So if biology is relevant to parental obligations— as it is—this is so only when certain additional conditions are met.

Biology can play a role in the generation of parental obligations even if they are not undertaken in the standard way, by deciding to procreate. Consider, for example, a case of failed contraception in which pregnancy results despite the partners having taken reasonable care to avoid conception. Suppose Marcia cannot bring herself to have an abortion or to put up the child for adoption, so she decides to have and raise the child. The father, Anthony, asserts that he has no obligations to this child, which he admits is his, because he never intended to become a father, indeed took steps to avoid becoming one, and has made it clear to the mother that she is on her own if she decides to go through with the pregnancy. He claims further that it would be unfair to expect him to support the child, that he should not be held hostage to the mother's unilateral decision.

One way to think about the biological father's parental obligations in this situation is to propose an analogy with the strict liability that is imputed to individuals who have unintentionally caused harm by foreseeably risky actions. Though the analogy is imperfect, it may nevertheless be close enough to suggest that Anthony is more than just the biological father. Though Anthony does not make someone worse off simply by participating in the creation of a child, the child will be harmed if he or she is not protected. By participating in the creation of this vulnerable human being, one might argue, Anthony incurs at least a prima facie obligation to prevent harm to the child. Here, biology plays an important role in generating Anthony's parental obligations, but only because two further conditions have been satisfied: he voluntarily engaged in sexual intercourse, and he knew, or should have known, that this carried a risk of resulting in a pregnancy.

Of course, Marcia could elect to have an abortion, and if she does, this would relieve her sexual partner of his parental obligations (although not necessarily of all obligations to Marcia). However, the decision to have an abortion ultimately rests with the woman, and she is not obligated to have an abortion even if she once told her partner that she would do so were she to become pregnant. She may change her mind. (By "change her mind" I mean to distinguish this from a case of deception. I say something about this below.) Thus Anthony should have known that if she became pregnant she might decide to keep the baby, and he cannot escape parental obligations by claiming, however sincerely, that he had assumed otherwise.

This is still not quite the complete story, however, for in determining whether biological parents have parental obligations, we also need to consider social child-rearing practices, conventions, and expectations. Elsewhere I have argued that assessing child-rearing arrangements involves determining how well they solve a certain coordination problem, namely, the problem of finding a coherent set of social practices that confer rights and duties that satisfy the interlocking interests of three distinct but interdependent parties: children (whose claims have some, but not absolute, priority), child rearers, and society at large (which also has legitimate interests in the procreation and raising of children) (Blustein 1982). Various child-rearing arrangements can be imagined, in some of which biological parents are not the normal child rearers, and these might be acceptable solutions to the coordination problem, even though the biological parents have very different obligations than they do under our society's current child-rearing arrangements. In the early days of the Israeli kibbutzim, for example, obligations to discipline and educate children, traditionally borne by biological parents, were undertaken by professional caretakers on behalf of the community at large. Further discussion of alternative child-rearing practices, however, would take me too far afield.

Though questions about the appropriate use of DNA-based identity testing may serve as a stepping-off place for challenging the basic structure of current child-rearing practices, more immediate concerns need to be addressed. I will suppose, therefore, that child-rearing practices in which biological parents have primary responsibility for their children, while perhaps not optimal from the standpoint of satisfying the three sets of interlocking interests, are among the acceptable alternatives.

Assuming, then, that biological parents normally have this responsibility, I propose the following principle:

> The Presumptive Connection between Biology and Parental Obligation: Because the conditions of voluntariness and reasonable foreknowledge are usually met, there are grounds for a presumption that the biological parent of a child has some parental obligations to that child.

This principle emphasizes the connection between procreation and the incurring of a moral obligation for the upbringing of a child. It does not assert a connection between the act of generation and the acquisition of a distinct parental right. I return to this important qualification later in the chapter.

This analysis is relevant to case III above, in which Francine requests DNA paternity testing to establish that Bob is the biological father and has support obligations because of this. The argument would run as follows. If Bob is the biological father, despite his denial, he cannot simply walk away from the child. Economic support is critically important to children, and it is unfair to the mother, and potentially detrimental to the child, to burden the mother with full responsibility for the child's support. Assuming that Bob voluntarily engaged in intercourse with the knowledge that a pregnancy might result and that he has the financial means to contribute to the child's support, there are solid grounds for requiring him to do so. (I assume further that he may not compel Francine to have an abortion or to give up the child for adoption.) The fact that Bob and Francine are not married and that he never led her to believe that he had a long-term commitment to her does not alter this conclusion. Marriage establishes a presumption that the husband of the biological mother is the biological father of her child, but the absence of marriage establishes no presumption in favor of the man who claims not to be the biological father of the child and to have no parental obligations. In the absence of good reasons to believe that Bob could not be the biological father of Francine's child, the DNA paternity test should be done.

It may be countered that whether paternity triggers economic responsibility depends on the structure of economic support available to children, and this depends on the particular family policy adopted by the society. Different policies have different implications for parents' economic responsibilities. Under a completely public system of economic support for children, biological fathers would have no obligations to pay support. Under a modified private system, by contrast, government would provide backup child support if support was not paid or was inadequate to meet the needs of children. In this arrangement, parental support obligations would not cease but would be supplemented by government support to ensure sufficient resources for children. Under a largely private system of child support, such as in the United States, economic support for children is chiefly the responsibility of individual parents.

Between a mixed private/public and a purely private system of child support, there are strong reasons for preferring the former, given that under the latter arrangement the financial circumstances of a significant number of children may be insufficient to meet their needs. However, the choice between a mixed private/public and a public system may be more complicated. Would a public system foster paternal irresponsibility and disconnection? Would it make matters worse overall for children? Or is a public system the only way to truly equalize opportunities for children? Though I cannot pursue these important questions of social policy here, I would argue that debates over the respective merits of public versus mixed private/public systems of child support are largely academic in U.S. society. Biological parents will continue to have economic obligations to their children because, in an individualistic society such as ours, a public system of child support is unlikely to achieve widespread acceptance.

I now want to introduce a complicating factor. In the case of Marcia and Anthony, there is no suggestion that she deceived him into believing she was using a contraceptive. However, it is not clear how, if at all, such deception would alter Anthony's parental obligations, given that he is still the biological father (he does not contest this) and intercourse is an inherently unpredictable activity even when contraceptives are used. Nonetheless, maternal deception may be alleged by the biological father as a way of relieving himself of parental obligations. This is different from the case in which maternal deception is alleged by the putative father with respect to his status as the biological father. If nonpaternity is established before or during a divorce proceeding, he may claim that he should not be forced to assume financial responsibility for children he was duped into believing were his own, children another man should be supporting.

The putative father's sense of unfairness is perhaps understandable: the biological father probably *should* be supporting his children. But what role should the mother's deception play in determining the putative father's child support obligations? One relevant consideration here is brought out in the two variants of case I above—that is, the availability of the biological father. If the biological father is available, then, as I argued in discussing the role of biology in the creation of parental obligations, there is a presumption that he has (at least) support obligations. Even then, there may be grounds for claiming that the putative father is not totally absolved of the obligation to pay financial support. But more troubling is the case where the biological father is not available. In this situation, the putative father might assert that imposing an obligation on him to pay child support for another man's child only compounds the initial wrong he suffered because of the deception, and therefore he should be relieved of this obligation. However, before we accept this argument, we need to look for other possible grounds of parental obligation.

Parental Obligations Arising from the Psychological Parent-Child Relationship

I claimed earlier that one standard way of acquiring parental obligations is to undertake them. Deciding to procreate is perhaps the most common way of undertaking these obligations. But, of course, one can undertake parental obligations even if one played no procreative role. Adoption, in which parental obligations are quite explicitly undertaken, is usually mentioned in this connection. I want to focus, however, on another sort of case, in which parental obligations are undertaken by a nonadoptive father who did not beget the child, although he might have undertaken these obligations because he (falsely) believed he was the biological father.

Let us continue with and expand on the discussion of Joe and Lynn in case I. Joe may not be the biological father of the child he has nurtured and cared for, but he has become what Goldstein, Freud, and Solnit (1973) call the *psychological* parent of this child. They explain this notion as follows: "Whether any adult becomes the psychological parent of a child is based on day-to-day interaction, companionship, and shared experiences. The role can be fulfilled either by a biological parent or by an adoptive parent or by any other caring adult—but never by an absent, inactive adult, whatever his biological or legal relationship to the child may be" (19). Joe has fulfilled this role not as a biological or adoptive parent but as a caring adult who made it known to the child—and not only to the child—that he or she can depend on him for guidance, protection, and love. He has undertaken the task of functioning as this child's psychological parent, daily renewing this commitment by his continuing companionship and support, and in so doing he has undertaken parental obligations. Suppose now that Joe and Lynn are getting a divorce, that Joe seeks to disestablish paternity so that he can be relieved of child support obligations, and that, if his suspicions of nonpaternity are confirmed, the actual biological father cannot be found or is in some other way unavailable to pay support (variant Ia). If the DNA test shows Joe not to be the biological father, should he be required to support the child? Perhaps on divorce he should have the choice either to maintain or to terminate the nonbiological father-child relationship. However, this view assumes that parental obligations are "a mere adjunct to the marriage, terminable with the end of the marriage" (Glennon 2000, 592), and it gives greater weight to the interests of the presumed father than to those of the still dependent child.

This is an ethically indefensible position. A different weighting of parents' and children's interests is reflected in the following principle:

Obligations Grounded in Psychological Parenting: Once parental obligations are undertaken by a person's becoming a child's psychological parent, they cannot be abrogated merely by a finding of nonpaternity.

The ability to provide financial support for a child's care and upbringing is something that prospective parents ought to consider, and financial support is one of the obligations parents incur. Joe's ongoing obligations to his child certainly encompass more than this, but according to this principle, his support obligations are not terminable on a finding of nonpaternity or on the dissolution of his marriage. Thus Joe may be obligated to pay support for another man's child if this is needed to safeguard the child's well-being. For the same reason, he may be obligated to share support obligations with the biological father, if the latter is available.

Against this there are two objections. First, one might argue that if a presumed father was unaware that he was not the biological father when he developed a psychological relationship with the child, then he did not *voluntarily* assume parental obligations, and it is unfair to place continued support obligations on someone under these conditions. Second, one might object that a presumed father's desire to discontinue child support after a finding of nonpaternity demonstrates that his psychological relationship with the child is not as close and loving as was assumed and, further, that we only cause more damage to the relationship by compelling him to continue paying child support. Neither of these objections is convincing, however. The acceptance of parental obligations over a long period of time is by itself sufficient evidence of voluntariness, and a nonbiological father's desire to be relieved of support obligations often says more about his relationship with the child's mother than that with the child. To be sure, if Joe has been wronged by his adulterous wife, the wrong should be properly addressed by the offending party: it should be acknowledged and forgiveness should be sought. But this is an issue to be worked out between Joe and Lynn and it does not affect the parental obligations Joe has incurred.

The theory of parenthood underlying this principle holds that parental obligations undertaken by procreation, adoption, or psychological parenting have a certain normative structure. That is, the interests of parents should be promoted and protected only if doing so is not inconsistent with the performance of parental responsibilities, so parents must adjust their individual needs and personal goals to the needs and legitimate interests of the children who are dependent on them. This child-centered conception of parenthood implies that, in the specific case under discussion, ensuring that a child continues to receive an adequate level of material support takes priority over the father's interest in avoiding support for another man's child. The principle also implies that in a situation such as case IV, a woman cannot use a finding of nonpaternity to sever the psychological bond between the nonbiological father and his child and prevent him from fulfilling his parental obligations.

The requirement that the pursuit of parental interests must not be inconsistent with the protection of children's interests does not preclude parents from having certain discretionary rights. Parental discretion in the upbringing of children is permissible as long as it is constrained by parental obligations to protect and promote the interests of those children. Thus reasonable parental discretion is allowed about how to fulfill parental obligations, but not about what obligations parents have. Moreover, parents are permitted to shape their children's lives according to the beliefs and values of the particular way of life to which the parents are committed, as long as in doing so they do not fail to fulfill their obligations to care for their children. Both sorts of parental discretion are morally permissible, and to this extent we can speak about parental *rights*. But one must be careful here. Emphasizing parental rights tends to focus attention on the interests of parents, whereas on the view I hold, the extent of permissible parental discretion is to be determined by reference to the welfare of children.

The principle that parental obligations, once undertaken by a psychological parent, are not nullified by a finding of nonpaternity does not apply to case II, however. Here, Carl is not the psychological parent of Eva's biological child, and he might not even be this child's biological father. So let us suppose that none of the three main ways of undertaking parental obligations—procreation, adoption, and prior patterns of caring—apply to Carl. Under these circumstances, Carl might offer to help support the child, but it is unclear on what basis we can establish that he has any parental obligations to this child. Having sexual relations with Eva can generate obligations for Carl to care for and support *his* biological child (if other conditions of voluntariness and reasonable foreknowledge are met), but I have not argued that simply being married to Eva is sufficient to generate obligations for Carl to care for or support *another man's* biological child. If the child's biological father is unavailable or unable to pay support, then arguably the state has the responsibility to fill the vacuum and provide some form of material assistance to Eva as needed.

Biological Parenthood and the Assertion of Parental Rights

The decision to engage in sexual intercourse entails responsibility for the reasonably foreseeable consequences that do, or may, follow from the voluntary actions that are the immediate object of the decision. Even when those engaging in sexual intercourse do not intend conception to occur, they cannot for this reason disavow responsibility if conception does ensue. But asserting that procreation (under the right conditions) gives rise to parental obligations is a very different matter from claiming that procreation entitles biological parents to distinct parental rights. In thinking about this issue, it is important to emphasize the qualified nature of parental rights in general. Rights that arise from procreation are not unconditional and do not chiefly exist to serve the interests of parents; rather, they chiefly serve the interests of children, and these take priority in determining what rights parents have or whether they have any rights at all. The connection between procreation and rights clearly fails to obtain in cases of abuse and the usual instances of neglect: procreators forfeit their custodial rights and their rights to direct the upbringing of their children in these extreme cases. The case to which I now turn, however—case V, and in particular the variant Vb—raises a somewhat different issue about the relationship between procreation and parental rights.

The rights parents typically have are diverse and numerous. A partial list includes the right to name the child, to determine the child's domicile, to have custody of the child, to bring up the child in the religion of one's choice or no religion at all, to direct and shape the child's psychological and social development, and to be obeyed by the child when he or she is young. There is also the expectation and possibly the right to receive honor and respect when obedience is no longer appropriate. Generally speaking, parental rights can be waived, delegated, forfeited, or otherwise lost, and specific rights may or may not be entailed by parental obligations. The parental right that I want to discuss in the context of DNA paternity testing is what might be called *the right to have and maintain a connection and relationship with the child* or, alternatively, the right to psychological parenthood.

Biological parents who are willing and able to care for and nurture their children usually do have this right, of course, and they can assert it against outside parties (including the state) to safeguard the integrity of the psychological parent-child relationship. However, as the following principle asserts, biology alone does not give the adult a right to establish and maintain a psychological relationship with the child:

> The Nonbiological Basis of Parental Rights: Paternity, while it may trigger economic responsibility in a private or mixed private/public system of child support, does not by itself give rise to rights of connection and relationship with the child.

Nancy E. Dowd (2000) argues the point this way: "Economic responsibility ought to be separated from the right to presence and access in order to disconnect [*sic*] the notion that children are property and that access can be bought . . . Economic responsibility ought to be grounded in a responsibility to life created and brought into this world, whereas rights of connection and relationship are grounded in care and nurture" (223). It follows, for example, that fathers who have chosen not to maintain a relationship with their children, but who later change their minds, cannot cite their payment of child support as sufficient basis for a right to psychological parenthood.

Let us turn now to case V. In variant Va, George seeks to establish his paternity shortly after the birth of the child so that he can have a relationship with the child. I would argue that, if George is willing to provide care and nurture and has planned for a future relationship with the child, he should not normally be barred from having this relationship or denied visitation. But in variant Vb, George's paternity is established several years after the child's birth, and during this time Jean's husband has become the child's psychological parent. George's motives for seeking a paternity test are not specified: he may have been motivated by revenge, by a deeply felt need to fill a void in his life, or by a genuine desire to provide guidance and support to his child. We need not attribute discreditable motives to him for failing to seek paternity testing earlier, and he might sincerely regret not having acted sooner. (Of course, his claim of parental rights might be weakened or defeated, depending on the reason for the delay.) But whether George now has rights of connection and relationship should his paternity be established does not depend only on his blameworthiness or his reasons for being tested. It depends also on what is good or at least not harmful for the child—that is, on whether George's establishing a relationship with the child at this point in his or her life is or is not detrimental to the child's psychological development and emotional well-being. Perhaps George should be given some preference over a non–biologically related stranger who wants to establish a relationship with the child. Nonetheless, if George's assertion of paternity and visitation rights would be seriously disruptive of the family unit and injurious to the child, then, paternity notwithstanding, this settles the matter as far as George's right to have a relationship with the child is concerned.

Restrictions on the Use of DNA Paternity Testing: Policy Considerations

For various reasons, the state may have a legitimate interest in determining biological/genetic parenthood. As E. Donald Shapiro and colleagues note, "succession rights, citizenship rights and medical necessities are just some of the reasons, other than support or tax obligations, that a state would want its citizenry properly defined by their biological relations" (Shapiro, Reifler, and Psome 1992–93, 26). But as we have seen, a number of issues need to be considered in deciding on the permissible use of DNA-based paternity information, including but not limited to determining biological parenthood for the purpose of imposing support obligations on reluctant fathers. A woman or her partner or both may seek paternity testing to deny the presumptive father of her child parental rights; a man may hope to prove paternity to assert parental rights of relationship with the child of a woman to whom he is not married or to disprove paternity so that he can relieve himself of parental obligations, even if the child's biological father is unavailable. The question I now want to ask is, what position should the state adopt toward paternity testing that individuals seek or undergo for these reasons? More narrowly, what is good public policy for determining when courts of law should allow the question of paternity to be raised and proof to be offered? Having answered these questions, we can then take up the issue of implementation; that is, we can consider resources and procedures that should be used to carry out the preferred policy.

There are, roughly speaking, three possible approaches to the narrower policy question, what I will call the never, always, and sometimes options.

Never. On this view, except in extremely rare circumstances, presumed fathers are not allowed to introduce evidence of nonpaternity, and men who are not married to the mother of the child in question are not allowed to introduce evidence of paternity to claim parental rights. The reasoning here is that the court's role is to protect the social institutions of marriage and family and that, for the sake the child's well-being, established parent-child relationships should not be disrupted.

Always. On this view, evidence of paternity or nonpaternity is always admissible in court. The reasoning behind this approach rests on claims of unfairness. That is, by allowing evidence of nonpaternity, we recognize the unfairness of requiring nonbiological fathers to pay support for a child who is not theirs, and by allowing evidence of paternity, we recognize the unfairness of imposing parental obligations on biological fathers without also permitting them to assert their paternity rights when they choose to do so. A further advantage of this approach, one might argue, is that policies allowing evidence of paternity would support biological fathers in their efforts to assume fathering responsibilities, which is something society ought to promote.

Sometimes. On this view, evidence of nonpaternity or paternity is sometimes admitted and sometimes not, depending on a number of factors. These include (1) the sort of relationship, if any, that has developed between the child and the presumed father; (2) the impact on the child of permitting the father whose paternity is established by DNA testing to assume a parental role; (3) the harm that may result to the child if presumed paternity is disproved; (4) the age of the child; and (5) the availability of the biological father and his ability to bear the financial costs of the child's upbringing.

It should be clear from my discussion thus far that I favor the third option. The "never" and "always" approaches strike the wrong balance between competing interests. The former neglects the interests of husbands and biological fathers in the name of upholding some idealized vision of marriage and family. The latter gives these interests overriding importance and also attempts to promote responsible fatherhood to the possible detriment of the child. The preferred approach steers a middle course between these extremes. It ranks the interests of the child above those of the husband and biological father, and it weighs the admissibility of evidence of paternity and nonpaternity according to how giving this legal force and allowing it to be litigated would affect the child's well-being. This policy recognizes that husbands and biological fathers may have legitimate interests worthy of acknowledgment and protection, and it permits these persons to give voice to them. But it gives priority to the state's *parens patriae* obligation to shield vulnerable children from the actions of parents and would-be parents that threaten their welfare.

Admittedly, the two extreme approaches do not require much in the way of individualized decision making, unlike the intermediate position, and this may be thought to count in their favor. Judges, it may be claimed, often lack the training and expertise to identify and properly weigh the diverse factors that need to be considered in deciding what effect, if any, information about paternity should have on parental obligations and rights. Moreover, if the intermediate approach were adopted, the argument continues, it would give individual judges too much discretion to impose their personal values in deciding whether to allow evidence of paternity to be raised and litigated, thus introducing subjective biases and uncritical assumptions about parents and children into the decision-making process. Clear, determinate, and easily applied rules, as represented by the "never" and "always" approaches, would leave little scope for bias and would permit consistency of decision making from case to case.

Even if we concede the last points, the "sometimes" approach is so clearly ethically preferable to the other two that we should ask whether we can find ways to meet these objections and strengthen the case for the intermediate position. I believe we can. Judges may indeed lack the training and expertise to resolve these complex issues, but the problem is not insurmountable. Mental health professionals, child development experts, and others can assist judges in making sound decisions by providing testimony about the harm that would or would not ensue to the parties (and especially the child) if the issue of paternity were litigated. Indeed, these professionals often do assist family and juvenile court judges in this way. Arguably their testimony should be incorporated into any judicial determination of admissibility as a safeguard against ill-informed and hasty decision making.

In addition, the flexibility in decision making required by the intermediate position can be built into the judicial process by annexing some sort of alternative dispute resolution process. Advocates of alternative dispute resolution claim that such methods have in common a number of characteristics that make them more suitable than litigation for a wide range of cases, including speedier resolution and greater openness, flexibility, and responsiveness to the needs of the individual participants. Mediation in particular is increasingly being used as an alternative to formal legal processes for the resolution of family issues, and this is an attractive option for resolving the complex issues surrounding the use of DNA-based paternity information. Judges can—and in many, perhaps most, cases should—order parties to go for mediation before coming to court, and can supervise the process.

In short, by using the expertise of psychologists and other professionals and alternative dispute resolution processes such as mediation, along with other measures, family and juvenile courts stand a reasonably good chance of achieving flexibility without sacrificing fairness. Moreover, it is hard to see why some other arrangement in which courts do not play a central role would be a better option in this respect. Of course, even the best approach will sometimes fail to adequately protect children and the rights and interests of other involved parties. But in matters as sensitive and complicated as these, perfection is not to be expected.

ACKNOWLEDGMENTS

I thank the Hon. Michael Gage, former Administrative Judge of the Family Court of the City of New York, for helpful discussion about law and policy.

BIBLIOGRAPHY

Blustein, J. 1982. *Parents and Children: The Ethics of the Family.* New York: Oxford University Press.

———. 1983. On the doctrine of parens patriae: Fiduciary obligations and state power. *Criminal Justice Ethics* 2:39–47.

———. 1997. Procreation and parental responsibility. *Journal of Social Philosophy* 28:79–86.

Dowd, N. E. 2000. *Redefining Fatherhood.* New York: New York University Press.

Glennon, T. 2000. Somebody's child: Evaluating the erosion of the marital presumption of paternity. *West Virginia Law Review* 102:547–605.

Goldstein, J., A. Freud, and A. J. Solnit. 1973. *Beyond the Best Interests of the Child.* New York: Free Press.

Kaplan, D. 2000. Why truth is not a defense in paternity actions. *Texas Journal of Women and the Law* 10:69–81.

Marchese, S. 2001. Putting square pegs into round holes: Mediation and the rights of children with disabilities under the IDEA. *Rutgers Law Review* 53:333–65.

Montague, P. 2000. The myth of parental rights. *Social Theory and Practice* 26:47–68.

O'Neill, O. 1979. Begetting, bearing, and rearing. In *Having Children,* ed. O. O'Neill and W. Ruddick, 25–38. New York: Oxford University Press.

Pruett, E., and C. Savage. 2004. Models of collaboration in family law: Statewide initiatives to encourage alternative dispute resolution and enhance collaborative approaches to resolving family issues. *Family Court Review* 42:232–43.

Riskin, L. L., and J. E. Westbrook. 1997. *Dispute Resolution and Lawyers,* 2nd ed. St. Paul, MN: West Publishing.

Robinson, B., and S. Paikin. 2001. Who is daddy? A case for the Uniform Parentage Act. *Delaware Lawyer* 19:23–27.

Shapiro, E. D., S. Reifler, and C. L. Psome. 1992–93. The DNA paternity test: Legislating the future paternity action. *Journal of Law and Health* 7:1–30.

Trakman, L. E. 2001. Appropriate conflict management. *Wisconsin Law Review* 2001: 919–29.

Zuberbuhler, J. 2001. Early intervention mediation: The use of court-ordered mediation in the initial stages of divorce litigation to resolve parenting issues. *Family Court Review* 39:203–6.

CHAPTER FOUR

Paternity Testing, Family Relationships, and Child Well-Being

Diane Scott-Jones, Ph.D.

Paternity testing must be considered in the context of parent-child relationships, other family relationships, and the social setting in which the family lives. Paternity testing is consequential for the father and for the children connected to that father, whether the connection is biological or social or both. Paternity testing may confirm or shatter an identity for the father as well as for the child whose parentage is in question. Paternity testing may disrupt family life. Siblings may learn they are half-siblings and new siblings may be discovered. Paternity testing may force financial support of a child or may relieve a putative father of the responsibility of child support. In this chapter I examine the issue of paternity testing from the perspective of psychology—particularly developmental psychology.

Developmental Perspective

In the United States, our cultural ideology orients us to think about the development of individuals. Children's lives and parents' lives, however, are intertwined with one another and with the life trajectories of other family members. The life course of a child unfolds in a complex network of mutually influencing social relationships. DNA paternity testing occurs in the context of these intertwined developmental pathways.

Children experience both normative and nonnormative life events throughout their development. Normative life events occur at a regular time and in a relatively similar manner for a wide range of children—examples are the beginning of formal schooling at five or six years of age and the onset of puberty in early adolescence. Normative events may be stressful, but families and other social institutions prepare children for these potentially stressful events. We develop cultural scripts and social supports for the normative events children experience. Nonnormative life events, such as parents' divorce or learning your father is not actually your biological father, are more problematic because they are unexpected; there is no preparation and no readily available cultural script.

Children's development is probabilistic, not lawful. We can identify family structures and family processes that increase the probability of adverse outcomes for children, but children can and do adapt successfully to a wide range of family arrangements. Children's outcomes are determined by many factors. Their social, emotional, and cognitive development is not typically determined by a single event. Children are resilient as well as fragile. Some children prosper despite negative life situations; some children fail to thrive in ostensibly positive environments.

Children are active and thinking in development; they construct meanings from their experiences and are not mere passive recipients of parental socialization. In addition to parents' affecting children, children's characteristics and behavior affect parents. Although parents are more powerful and more responsible than children in the process of socialization, bidirectional influences occur throughout development, beginning in infancy (Bell 1968, 1979).

Our research methods in developmental psychology orient us to assess group differences, and we give insufficient attention to within-group variability. Yet much variation occurs among children grouped by any social category—including family structure (parents divorced, not divorced; biological father present, biological father absent) and other social categories such as socioeconomic status, gender, and ethnic background.

Children develop in a relational context, typically in a family. That family context, in turn, is grounded in a sociohistorical context. The broader social context influences the way in which children and adult family members interpret their own lives. For example, the prevalence of divorce in a society influences the way in which children experience and understand marital disruptions in their own families.

Some methodological issues are challenges in the field of developmental psychology. We should consider DNA paternity testing in a relational context;

however, much psychological research relies on assessments of single individuals instead of individuals in a relational context. Many studies rely on one individual reporting the behavior of another, such as a mother's reports of her child's behavior, or one individual describing family interactions, such as an adolescent reporting his or her relationship with parents. Some studies assess dyadic interactions, such as mother and child or husband and wife interacting together, and a few assess more than two family members interacting. Studies that actually assess family members in a relational context are difficult to conduct. The hallmark of developmental research is the longitudinal study, which provides more than a single picture of family interactions at one point in time, but we have only a few major studies that follow the course of family relationships through disruption, divorce, and remarriage over time.

Studies of varied family arrangements and family events may be based on an implicit conception of an "ideal family" that does not fit actual families now or in the past. The circumstances surrounding DNA paternity testing often are compared with an ideal family situation instead of variations around that ideal, such as families experiencing divorce.

Contexts of DNA Paternity Testing

The family context and sociohistorical context in which paternity is established or contested are important. The case of Morgan Wise (Lewin 2001) has been widely discussed. An examination of the situation of the Wise family reveals substantial family problems and nonnormative life events, in addition to the misattributed paternity. Any one of these problems, or nonnormative events, could have contributed to vulnerabilities in the children and adults in this family before the problem of misattributed paternity arose.

Divorce. The parents were divorced. Half of all marriages in the United States end in divorce, but cultural scripts to explain divorce are lacking, and strategies for adjustment of children and adults following divorce are not clear cut. Divorce has become so common, however, that terms such as "serial monogamy," "progressive monogamy," and "serial marriage" have been used to refer to the marital arrangements in U.S. society (Brody, Neubaum, and Forehand 1988). Divorce may one day become a normative life event, instead of a nonnormative event, for adults and children, but for now, divorce is disruptive for children and adults and requires a period of adjustment.

Father custody. Following the divorce, the father, Morgan Wise, took custody of his children. Although custody decisions should be gender neutral, mothers typically are granted custody of their children. The proportion of single-father families in the United States has increased from 1 percent of families in 1970 to 5 percent in 2000 (Fields and Casper 2001), but single-father families still are rare.

Integrating family and work. Morgan Wise experienced problems integrating his work life with his family life as a divorced custodial father. Multiple roles in the family and at work are beneficial to men and women, except when the demands of one or more roles are excessive and lead to overload and distress (Barnett and Hyde 2001). As a single father and a railroad engineer, Wise found caring for his four children difficult. Because of the demands of his work, the Wise children experienced an additional disruption—a change from paternal custody to maternal custody. Transitions such as moving from one household to another are associated with adjustment problems in children (Adam and Chase-Lansdale 2002).

Chronic and serious childhood illness. The Wise family experienced the problems of a chronic childhood illness—cystic fibrosis. Even in the best of family circumstances, managing a chronic childhood illness is difficult for parents as well as for the ill child, the siblings, and members of the extended family. Married couples who have a child with cystic fibrosis report greater role strain and less time in recreational activities than couples with a healthy child (Quittner et al. 1992).

Added to these problems was the discovery, based on DNA evidence, that the social father, Morgan Wise, was not the biological father of three of his four children. This fact was uncovered in an emotionally charged family situation, during tests related to the son's treatment for cystic fibrosis. A complex web of family relationships and several family problems existed before the test results that raised questions about the children's biological father. The DNA test results changed the father's understanding of his relationship to his children and his relationship with the children's mother. Betrayal and deception in the marital relationship became evident. Despite the DNA evidence, Wise was not relieved of his legal obligations for child support, and the U.S. Supreme Court in 2002 refused to hear his case (*Wise v. Fryar* 2002).

Historically, other instances of contested or unclaimed paternity have occurred, but social fathers and other adults often have reared children successfully in these cases of misattributed paternity. American society also has maintained secrecy about biological fatherhood in socially taboo relationships. A well-known example is Thomas Jefferson's alleged fathering of the children of Sally Hemings, who was a slave (Gordon-Reed 1997; Woodson 2001). That biological relationship now has some support, albeit ambiguous, from DNA testing of descendants and alleged descendants. More recently, after the death of segregationist Senator Strom Thurmond at one hundred years of age, his seventy-eight-year-old first-born but unacknowledged daughter revealed publicly that her biological parents were Thurmond and Carrie Butler, an African American woman who was sixteen years of age at the time of the birth (Foston 2004). Other less celebrated or less notorious instances of unclaimed or unacknowledged fatherhood have become known as African American persons search for their Caucasian ancestors (e.g., Henry 2001). Our society has shown a remarkable capacity for maintaining social fictions about biological fatherhood. Social power was a key element in misattributed paternity. With powerful biological fathers and relatively powerless mothers, the child's biological lineage and social location were misrepresented. In many of these cases, families now are seeking information about biological paternity because they wish to right a social wrong and correct the historical and biological record, not because social fathers were inadequate in child rearing.

Fathers and Children

All cultures recognize the social role of father, although other male kin, instead of the biological father, may routinely take or share the paternal role (Engle and Breaux 1998). Our use of language, however, supports an emphasis on the biology of fatherhood and on the social relationship of motherhood. *To father* a child typically refers to the biological act of procreation, whereas *mothering* or *to mother* typically refers to acts of nurturing. To father is "to beget" or produce offspring. To mother is "to care for or protect." Social changes in divorce and remarriage are forcing a movement away from completely biological definitions of *father* to broader definitions that recognize that fathers can be social or biological or both and can be legal or nonlegal (Tamis-LeMonda and Cabrera 1999). For example, a stepfather may be an actively involved social father but will have no legal rights or legal responsibilities unless he adopts his stepchildren. Further, with urbanization and with women working outside the home in many cultures, there is an increasing expectation that fathers will be actively involved with their children in a nurturing role in addition to the traditional economic role (Engle and Breaux 1998).

Research on fathers is increasing, but fathers have been understudied in developmental psychology. Fathers' roles in the family and in child rearing are often reported by mothers. Studies of parenting are often studies of mothers only, not fathers. Even major recent works on parent-offspring attachment (e.g., Crittenden and Claussen 2000) focus on mothers and children. Attention is given to fathers when they are absent from the formal, recognized family. Studies of divorce and single parenthood still focus mainly on women and children.

Generativity—Psychological and Biological

Snarey and colleagues have reported a longitudinal study of fathers that spans four decades (Snarey 1993; Snarey et al. 1987). Fathers were interviewed about their sons and daughters; these fathers had been interviewed when they were boys, about their own parents. The 343 participating fathers were Caucasian, born in urban communities in Boston during the Great Depression, and most were poor during boyhood. These fathers' offspring are part of the baby boom generation.

The study was based on Erik Erikson's theory, which assumes a series of psychosocial stages throughout the life span, with middle adulthood marked by a concern for contributing to the next generation. Men, like women, feel a sense of achievement with the birth of a child. In Erikson's theory, this sense of accomplishment with the conception, birth, and first-year care of offspring is referred to as *biological generativity. Psychological generativity,* in contrast to stagnation or self-absorption, is caring that contributes to future generations. Psychological generativity includes child rearing as well as social and cultural contributions outside the biological family.

Snarey and colleagues found that children had great significance for fathers' psychosocial development, that fathers' involvement in child rearing was positively associated with their children's adult outcomes, and that fathers became better at parenting and more involved than their own fathers were. In the conceptual framework of this study, infertility or reproductive difficulty is a threat to generativity and, according to Snarey, is indirectly a threat to social and cultural generativity. Of the men in the study, 15 percent had infertility problems. Some became involved in activities with other children and later adopted a child. The men who experienced infertility but later adopted were more highly involved in child rearing than were men who became biological fathers without any problems.

Similarly, Golombok and coauthors reported that fathers in families that used assisted conception (including donor gametes and in vitro fertilization) interacted more with their four- to eight-year-old children than did "natural" fathers (Golombok et al. 1995; Golombok 1999). Evolutionary and biological theories posit that fathers invest more when they are genetically related to their children and are certain of the genetic relationship, but support for this view of the primacy of biological relatedness is equivocal (Engle and Breaux 1998). Clearly, social fathers establish ties with their children in the absence of a biological relationship.

Father-Child Interactions

Historical trends reveal more interactions of fathers with children currently than in the past. The contemporary ideal is the involved father, but there is much variation among families, with some retaining a traditional division of roles between mother and father and thus a limited paternal involvement. Attachment to infants, however, occurs for fathers as well as for mothers (Belsky 1996), and observational studies indicate fathers and mothers are equally competent as early caregivers (Parke and Stearns 1993). With new family types, such as stepfamilies and recombined families, following divorce and remarriage, fathers are expected to be involved in children's lives even in the absence of a biological relationship (Tamis-LeMonda and Cabrera 1999).

Studies of the effects of parental acceptance and rejection of children on outcomes during childhood and adulthood in a wide range of cultural settings find, as one might expect, positive outcomes associated with acceptance (nurturance, affection, and support) and negative outcomes associated with rejection (absence or withdrawal of nurturance, affection, and support) (Rohner 1998). Most of the research has been conducted with mothers, but research on fathers finds that father's acceptance is often as strongly associated with positive child outcomes (cognitive and social competence, psychological adjustment) as is mother's acceptance; further, father's acceptance is sometimes more strongly associated with some outcomes than is mother's acceptance. According to Rohner, the positive role of father's acceptance has been ignored until recently because of widely held beliefs about the importance of mothers.

Work Commitment

In some periods in our past, men had more responsibility and more authority in child rearing than they do today. In colonial days and early in U.S. history, in the seventeenth and eighteenth centuries, husbands exerted control over wives and children, with or without the help of servants or slaves. Economic and social change, with the male workplace moving away from the home, led to the ideal of mothers as primary caretakers (Berry 1993). Fathers' work and financial support are important to children's well-being, but the demands of fathers' work may conflict with father-child interaction. Some studies found that the greater the salience or importance of his job to a father, the less involved that father was in child-care activities. Evidence is mixed on the possibilities of active paternal involvement in child rearing, although institutional support for fathers has increased (Parke and Stearns 1993). Men earn more than women, so the emphasis on fathers' economic role has some basis in gender differences in income. Fathers' economic role still looms large.

Financial Support

The primacy of fathers' biological role and their concomitant economic obligations have led to a lesser emphasis on the nurturing or social role of fathers. Social policies have tended to "slight fathers" and focus mainly on fathers' financial contributions to their children (Tamis-LeMonda and Cabrera 1999, 3). The instances of misattribution of paternity might be less disruptive and less painful if social policy emphasized the irreversible obligation of the social father to the child. Yet, whatever confusion may exist about biological fatherhood, financial support is critical to a child's well-being. Studies of single-parent families (e.g., McLanahan and Sandefur 1994) clearly call for greater efforts to require fathers to meet their financial obligations to children. Policies regarding mistaken paternity must incorporate the secure financial support of the child as a primary concern. This financial support is likely to be problematic, given the difficulties in American society in enforcing biological fathers' child support obligations.

The Child's Experiences and Perspectives

Do children experience more positive developmental outcomes when reared in a family in which they are biologically related to the social father? Research on adopted children and on children conceived by assisted reproduction may shed some light on the possible impact of having a social father who is not the biological father.

Children's understanding of their social worlds, kinship, and family relationships becomes more complex with age. As they mature, children's perspectives on their families become more realistic and sometimes more negative (Reid, Ramey, and Burchinal 1990). Disclosure to children is a key issue in cases of misattributed paternity. Secrecy and disclosure to children in families created through adoption and through assisted reproduction may provide models for handling the issues of secrecy and disclosure to children in cases of misattributed paternity.

Biological Fathers, Nonbiological Fathers, and Children's Outcomes

Some studies of adopted children suggest that parenting is difficult in the absence of a biological relationship between parent and child. Studies of adoption, like studies of divorce and single parenthood, need to take into account many other variables, such as family socioeconomic status and the child's age, that affect child outcomes. Some researchers use statistical controls for these variables, but research is needed that examines multiple variables simultaneously.

Research comparing adoptive families and families created with various forms of assisted reproduction suggests no significant differences in children's psychological well-being, parent-child interactions, and quality of parenting between genetically related and unrelated parents and children (Golombok et al. 1995; Golombok et al. 1999). Parents' psychological well-being, however, seems to differ. In a comparison of families using adoption, donor insemination, egg donation, or in vitro fertilization (IVF) with the parents' gametes, Golombok and colleagues (1999) reported the surprising finding that mothers' and fathers' psychological well-being was greater in families in which the mother was not genetically related to the child, regardless of the father's relationship to the child. The authors suggest that the greater psychological well-being may result from the parents' having a stronger desire to have a child when the mother is unable to conceive "naturally"; the strong desire for a child may be more closely related to well-being than are any factors associated with genetic links between parent and child. This interpretation is plausible but speculative and should be examined in empirical research. In addition to studies of group differences, studies are needed to assess and describe the process of adaptation in families using assisted reproductive technologies.

In a follow-up study when the children had reached twelve years of age, Golombok, MacCallum, and Goodman (2001) found that children conceived by in vitro fertilization (with parents' gametes, thus genetically related to both parents) seemed to be well-functioning and did not differ in socioemotional adjustment from adopted or naturally conceived children. A separate report (Golombok et al. 2002) compared the donor insemination (DI), adopted, and naturally conceived twelve-year-old children in the same longitudinal study. Children conceived by donor insemination were not more likely to show psychological disorders than were the adopted and naturally conceived children. The DI children also did not differ from the other two groups in self-reported peer relationships and adjustment to school. These findings of normal development in twelve-year-old IVF and DI children are important because the early adolescent years are sometimes marked by conflict with parents and by increased attention to identity.

In the longitudinal study (Golombok, MacCallum, and Goodman 2001; Golombok et al. 2002), mothers and fathers were assessed on two widely used parenting constructs: warmth and control. Overall, the IVF (genetically related to both parents), adoptive (in infancy), and naturally conceived families differed on warmth variables. Both mothers and fathers of children conceived by IVF showed greater warmth to their children (rated by interviewer) than did adoptive mothers and fathers but were not different in warmth from mothers and fathers of naturally conceived children. No differences were found for most of the nineteen variables assessing parental control (Golombok, MacCallum, and Goodman 2001). Fathers of children conceived by donor insemination had a high level of involvement in parenting, despite their having no genetic relationship with their child. These findings suggest that genetic ties are not necessary to fathers' positive relationships with the children they raise (Golombok et al. 2002).

Secrecy and Disclosure about Biological Fatherhood

Adoption is a family-building process for which we have developed cultural stories or cultural scripts to explain the process to the adopted child. Parents may be unable to have a biological child: a normative (i.e., regular or typical) life event thus becomes nonnormative. Or prospective parents may choose adoption because they are without partners with whom to have a child. In the past, adoption was shrouded in secrecy, and telling adopted children about their biological origins was not recommended. Openness, in contrast to secrecy, is currently thought to be associated with positive child and parental outcomes in adoptive families (Mendenhall, Grotevant, and McRoy 1996).

The meanings that parents, children, and others construct about the adoption process are likely to be important to the well-being of the family. Some researchers have investigated the stories or narratives that families create about themselves. In the Minnesota/Texas Adoption Research Project, couples in fully disclosed adoptions—those with ongoing, fully identified communication between the birth mother and the adoptive family—have more coherent narratives when asked to describe their experience of adoption (Grotevant et al. 1999). It is of interest that Grotevant and colleagues define *openness* in communication with the birth mother; there is no mention of the birth father in this study. The least coherent narratives came from families involved in confidential adoptions, in which there is no communication with the birth mother after placement of the child.

As noted above, society has socially acceptable stories to explain adoption to children (Golombok 1999). Standard children's storybooks are available to help parents create a family story for their adopted children. Beautifully written and illustrated, stories for young children are overwhelmingly positive about the adoption process. These stories include a gentle reference to the fact that the social mother could not "grow a baby"; perhaps the birth mother was too young to take care of the baby, and she was sad she could not keep her child. Overall, these stories convey the message that the adopted child is special and "chosen." Stories for older children present mild conflicts, which are resolved in a positive manner. For example, a boy realizes he does not look like the parents and wonders whether he did something wrong that caused his birth mother not to want to keep him. In one story, a school counselor helps the child feel better; another story emphasizes the permanence of adoption. Some of the stories that present a conflict involve the adoption of a Korean child or a Chinese child into a Caucasian American family. These stories emphasize the birth mother but not the birth father. The children's book *Are You My Mother?* uses animals to convey the notion that offspring should resemble their mother; in this engaging book about the persistent and thorough search for a mother, there is no reference to fathers at all. (See the appendix for a listing of children's books on these topics.)

The concept of "genealogical bewilderment" has been used to describe the assumed negative emotional response of a person who does not know his or her genetic forebears. In their counseling of DI couples, Humphrey and Humphrey (1986) reported that all the couples they counseled intended to keep the child's origins secret from the child, although almost half the couples had confided in their parents, siblings, and friends. The issue of secrecy versus disclosure is similar in adoption and in assisted reproduction. Based mainly on a review of the literature on adoption, Humphrey and Humphrey concluded that persons with a compulsion to search for their biological relatives were typically suffering from emotional deprivation or some adverse experience. They concluded that three factors are important when making decisions about disclosing information to the child: how much information is available to the adoptive parents, the quality and quantity of that information, and the timing of disclosure. Humphrey and Humphrey concluded that the long-term impact of uncertainty about genetic origins is dwarfed by the strong effects of positive family relationships.

Parents' stories about donor insemination reported by Rumball and Adair (1999) are much like adoption stories. The themes are similar: parental difficulty in having a baby, but with the focus on the father's "seeds" instead of the mother's inability to grow a child; strong parental desire for a child and sadness without a child; and the adopted child being a special child. Sometimes the well-planned stories backfire. Rumball and Adair described a mother whose child completely rejected her story that he had one mother and two fathers. This mother said she would try again and, next time, would describe the "donor" rather than the "second father."

Cook and co-workers (1995) conducted a study comparing disclosure about children's origins among parents using donor insemination, in vitro fertilization with parental gametes, and adoption. They found that the parents in the DI group were much less likely to disclose their child's origins to them than were adoptive parents or parents of children conceived by IVF with the parents' own gametes. None of the DI parents had disclosed this information to their children, who were four to eight years of age at the time of the study. A high percentage of the DI parents (80%) reported having made a definite decision not to tell the children. In sharp contrast, 81 percent of parents of children conceived by IVF with parents' gametes had already told (27%) or planned to tell (54%) the children. In the adoptive families, parents had told all but one of the fifty-five adopted children about their origins. All adoptive parents and almost all IVF parents had told family and friends about their children's origins. In contrast, almost half the DI parents had not told either the maternal or the paternal grandparents about their method of conception, and two-thirds had not told any of their friends. The percentage who had told maternal grandparents (51%) was more than twice the percentage who had told paternal grandparents (21%).

One of the major reasons for keeping donor insemination a secret was concern about possible negative reactions to the father's infertility from relatives and friends. Cook and colleagues (1995) suggested that general attitudes toward male infertility may be akin to those toward male sexual inadequacy or impotence. A second major reason for secrecy about donor insemination was the absence of guidance on the timing, content, and method of disclosure to children. The social norms and professional recommendations regarding disclosure to children differ greatly for parents using assisted reproductive technologies and for adoptive parents. In Cook and colleagues' study, all the adoptive parents reported that social workers/social services had advised or required them to tell their children they were adopted. In contrast, none of the IVF parents and only two of the forty-five DI parents reported getting any advice on disclosure to children from the clinics that provided their treatments. Adoptive parents described children's books that they used to help explain their children's origins, although these parents noted that the disclosure is much easier in the storybooks than in real life. Nevertheless, although difficulties might occur, the adoptive parents have "scripts" available in these storybooks to ease the burden of disclosure. Only a few children's storybooks are available to provide scripts for explaining assisted reproductive techniques. (See the appendix.)

In Cook and colleagues' study (1995), the third major problem that prevented parents' disclosure to DI children about their conception was that they had no genetic information to give their children about their biological fathers. Adoptive parents reported that they used information about the biological parents, including pictures in some cases, to explain adoption to their children. For IVF parents who used their own gametes, the issue of genetic relatedness does not occur. The DI parents did not have access to any information about the sperm donor.

The actual stories of donor insemination and assisted reproduction are more complex than merely recounting the basic biological facts. The story of genetic fatherhood and motherhood is likely to be wrapped up in conflicted family situations. Baran and Pannor (1989) recommend openness about donor insemination but the timing of disclosure may be important. Interviews with persons whose parents used donor insemination suggest that disclosure during adolescence may be problematic. Although these individuals adjusted to their life circumstances, they experienced considerable pain, not only from the fact of donor insemination but from conflict in their families. Respondents in Baran and Pannor's interviews often learned that their social father was not their biological father during an emotionally charged crisis. It is worth noting that some interviewees reported being relieved to learn their social father was not their biological father.

Few parents had disclosed assisted reproduction to their children in Golombok and colleagues' study (1999). None of the forty-five DI participants and only one of twenty-one egg donation participants had disclosed to their children, then four to eight years of age. In contrast, all fifty-five adoptive families had disclosed to their children, even though these children were adopted at six months or younger and were of the same ethnic background as their parents, and maintaining secrecy might have been possible.

Golombok and colleagues (1999) noted that openness may not always be better than secrecy; in their study, secrecy did not seem to have an adverse effect on the children, all eight years old or younger. These authors acknowledged that secrecy may lead to problems for these children later, especially because half of the DI parents and three-fourths of the egg donation parents had disclosed the use of donated gametes to persons other than their children and these individuals might tell the children about the assisted reproduction. Golombok and co-workers noted that the strongest commitment to secrecy occurred in families where the father did not have a genetic relationship with the child.

Secrecy in families created by assisted reproduction can lead to emotional difficulties, parent-child conflict, and identity confusion in children; some parents, however, may opt for secrecy because of the stigma of infertility (Golombok 1999). Problems may arise for children conceived by assisted reproduction once they reach adolescence, a time when parent-child conflict may occur and identity issues become salient for adolescents generally. In the follow-up study, when the children were twelve years of age, Golombok, MacCallum, and Goodman (2001) found that the majority of the parents (twenty-six of thirty-four families) had told their children they were conceived by IVF (with parents' gametes), four families planned to tell in the future, one family was unsure, and three families had decided not to tell. In contrast, only two of the thirty-seven children conceived by donor insemination had been told by twelve years of age (Golombok et al. 2002). As was true for these children at eight years of age, secrecy did not seem to have identifiable adverse consequences for the twelve-year-old children. Some parents reported regret that they had not told their children that their social father was not their biological father but felt that twelve years of age was too late to tell them. Again, problems might lie ahead if the children learn about their biological origins from individuals in whom their parents confided or from medical professionals when they undergo tests or treatments (Golombok et al. 2002).

Disclosure of adoption and assisted reproduction to children may remain problematic for future parents who use these strategies for creating their families. In a study of college students' attitudes toward adoption, assisted reproduction, and disclosure to children, the majority of participants favored disclosure of birth history to children but rated reactive disclosure (answering children's questions when asked) more highly than proactive disclosure (initiating discussion with children). Further, the majority of participants in this study reported they would disclose the use of assisted reproduction after the child reached ten years of age but would disclose adoption before ten years of age (Weiss et al. 2004).

Disclosure of Misattributed Paternity to Children

From a child's perspective, how different is learning about misattributed paternity from other kinds of disclosures about biological origins? As described above, explaining the details of conception and reproduction to children would seem to increase in difficulty from adoption, which is relatively easy to explain and could put parents in a positive, altruistic light; to IVF with parents' gametes, which, despite the past "test tube baby" label, still maintains the genetic connection between parents and offspring; to donor insemination and ovum donation, in which one or both parents may have no genetic relationship to the child. To add to the difficulty, explanations of misattributed paternity would require at least some reference to parental deception or lack of knowledge about sexual partners. Age would make a difference in whether the child could understand the deception involved in the marital relationship.

Considerations for DNA Paternity Testing

The current cultural construction of family, as well as the legal system, favors biological ties over emotional ties (Cherlin and Furstenberg 1994). The existence of more than two parents complicates the family system and the legal system, but the traditional idea of "family" is being replaced by more diverse constructions of family. The achieved or earned aspects of family ties should be considered as important as the ascribed or biological family relationships. The social ties that fathers establish with children remain important even if the biological relationship is found not to exist. As noted at the beginning of this chapter, children are both fragile and resilient in the face of family disruptions. Children's interests and concerns should remain at the forefront of decisions about family obligations. Presented here are four guidelines for policy.

Fathers generally play an important social role in child rearing. There is great variability, however, among fathers, and the current idealized notion of active paternal involvement is not achieved for all fathers. Because fathers' active involvement is generally associated with positive outcomes in children, policies should support the active involvement of social fathers—whether biological or not—in their children's lives. A child-rearing father, as much as a birth father, is obligated to make an irreversible commitment: social fathers and mothers have irreversible obligations to their children. The social aspects of fathering should be protected and encouraged, even when a social father learns he is not a biological father. Unfortunately, the social aspects of fathering are not as easy to regulate and enforce as are the financial responsibilities of being a father.

Reliable financial support is key to children's well-being. The child's need for this support throughout childhood should outweigh other concerns. DNA paternity testing should be used to establish support for a child, not to remove that support once it has begun. The case of Morgan Wise and other instances of misattributed paternity, such as *Paternity of Cheryl* (2001), have resulted in decisions that required men with established father-child relationships to continue financial support of the children not biologically their own. In *Cheryl,* the court's reasoning was that reversing a paternity judgment after five years could be devastating to the child, both emotionally and financially, and that the child's interests outweighed the father's interests. Policies regarding misattributed paternity should be administered in a way that acknowledges the elements of unfairness in the nonbiological, social fathers' situation, in addition to guaranteeing financial support of the child. For example, a newly identified biological father could be required to add his financial support of the child to that of the social father.

A child's well-being following disclosure of uncertainty or deception about his or her biological father will depend on many other aspects of family relationships, family processes, and characteristics of the child such as age and developmental level. Many children now grow up in complex family constellations, with a combination of biologically related and unrelated family members. In these complex families, children may become aware that the relationship between their biological mother and father has changed and that another man or woman has entered their mother's or father's life.

A child's understanding and acceptance of facts about biological paternity may change over time. Issues may emerge in adolescence and adulthood that were not of concern to the child. Some individuals may have a strong desire to find and establish relationships with biological fathers. Others may choose not to invest in finding an unknown biological father. Persons making either choice may be well-adjusted or poorly adjusted. Some specific needs, such as medical conditions, may lead a child to seek a biological father.

These guidelines for policy would help to protect children's well-being as social and legal institutions sort through the complexities that arise when DNA paternity testing reveals that social fathers are not biological fathers of their children. Children and adolescents need stable, caring social relationships with adults, and they need financial support. A strong social and economic foundation will help children and adolescents achieve positive developmental outcomes when they grow up in complex and changing family structures.

APPENDIX: CHILDREN'S BOOKS ON ADOPTION
AND ASSISTED REPRODUCTION

Adoption

Cole, J. *How I Was Adopted: Samantha's Story.* New York: Morrow Junior Books, 1995.
Curtis, J. L. *Tell Me Again about the Night I Was Born.* New York: Joanna Cotler Books, 1996.

Girard, L. W. *Adoption Is for Always*. Morton Grove, IL: Albert Whitman, 1986.

————. *We Adopted You, Benjamin Koo*. Morton Grove, IL: Albert Whitman, 1989.

McCutcheon, J. *Happy Adoption Day*. Boston: Little, Brown, 1996.

Peacock, C. A. *Mommy Far, Mommy Near*. Morton Grove, IL: Albert Whitman, 2000.

Assisted Reproduction

Appleton, T. *"I'm a Little Frostie,"* 2nd ed. Cambridge, UK: IFC Resource Centre, 1999.

————. *My Beginnings: A Very Special Story,* 2nd ed. Cambridge, UK: IFC Resource Centre, 1999.

Gordon, E. R. *Mommy Did I Grow in Your Tummy?* Santa Monica, CA: E. M. Greenberg Press, 1992.

Newman, L. *Heather Has Two Mommies,* 2nd ed. Los Angeles: Alyson Publications, 2000.

Schnitter, J. T. *Let Me Explain*. Indianapolis: Perspectives Press, 1995.

BIBLIOGRAPHY

Adam, E. K., and P. L. Chase-Lansdale. 2002. Home sweet home(s): Parental separations, residential moves, and adjustment problems in low-income adolescent girls. *Developmental Psychology* 38:792–805.

Baran, A., and R. Pannor. 1989. *Lethal Secrets: The Shocking Consequences of Unsolved Problems of Artificial Insemination*. New York: Warner Books.

Barnett, R. C., and J. S. Hyde. 2001. Women, men, work, and family: An expansionist theory. *American Psychologist* 56:781–96.

Bell, R. Q. 1968. A reinterpretation of the direction of effects in studies of socialization. *Psychological Review* 75:81–95.

————. 1979. Parent, child, and reciprocal influences. *American Psychologist* 34:821–26.

Belsky, J. 1996. Parent, infant, and social-contextual antecedents of father-son attachment security. *Developmental Psychology* 32:905–13.

Berry, M. F. 1993. *The Politics of Parenthood: Child Care, Women's Rights, and the Myth of the Good Mother*. New York: Penguin Books.

Brody, G. H., E. Neubaum, and R. Forehand. 1988. Serial marriage: A heuristic analysis of an emerging family form. *Psychological Bulletin* 103:211–22.

Cherlin, A. J., and F. F. Furstenberg, Jr. 1994. Step families in the United States: A reconsideration. *Annual Review of Sociology* 20:359–81.

Cook, R., S. Golombok, A. Bish, and C. Murray. 1995. Disclosure of donor insemination: Parental attitudes. *American Journal of Orthopsychiatry* 65:549–59.

Coontz, S. 1992. *The Way We Never Were: American Families and the Nostalgia Trap*. New York: Basic Books.

Crittenden, P. M., and A. H. Claussen, eds. 2000. *The Organization of Attachment Relationships: Maturation, Culture, and Context*. Cambridge: Cambridge University Press.

Engle, P. L., and C. Breaux. 1998. Father's involvement with children: Perspectives from developing countries. *Society for Research in Child Development Social Policy Report* 12:1–23.

Fields, J., and L. M. Casper. 2001. America's families and living arrangements, March 2000. *Current Population Reports*, no. P20-537. Washington, DC: U.S. Census Bureau.

Foston, N. A. 2004. Strom Thurmond's black family. *Ebony Magazine* 59:162, 164–66.

Golombok, S. 1999. New family forms: Children raised in solo mother families, lesbian mother families, and in families created by assisted reproduction. In *Child Psychology: A Handbook of Contemporary Issues*, ed. L. Balter and C. S. Tamis-LeMonda. Philadelphia: Psychology Press.

Golombok, S., R. Cook, A. Bish, and C. Murray. 1995. Families created by the new reproductive technologies: Quality of parenting and social and emotional development of the children. *Child Development* 66:285–98.

Golombok, S., F. MacCallum, and E. Goodman. 2001. The "test-tube" generation: Parent-child relationships and the psychological well-being of IVF children at adolescence. *Child Development* 72:599–608.

Golombok, S., F. MacCallum, E. Goodman, and M. Rutter. 2002. Families with children conceived by donor insemination: A follow-up at age 12. *Child Development* 73: 952–68.

Golombok, S., C. Murray, P. Brinsden, and H. Abdalla. 1999. Social versus biological parenting: Family functioning and the socioemotional development of children conceived by egg or sperm donation. *Journal of Child Psychology and Psychiatry* 40: 519–27.

Gordon-Reed, A. 1997. *Thomas Jefferson and Sally Hemings: An American Controversy.* Charlottesville: University Press of Virginia.

Grotevant, H. D., D. L. Fravel, D. Gorall, and J. Piper. 1999. Narratives of adoptive parents: Perspectives from individual and couple interviews. In *The Stories that Families Tell: Narrative Coherence, Narrative Interaction, and Relationship Beliefs*, vol. 64 of *Monographs of the Society for Research in Child Development*, ed. B. H. Fiese, A. J. Sameroff, H. D. Grotevant, F. S. Wamboldt, S. Dickstein, and D. L. Fravel, 69–83. Malden, MA: Blackwell.

Henry, N. 2001. *Pearl's Secret: A Black Man's Search for His White Family.* Berkeley and Los Angeles: University of California Press.

Humphrey, M., and H. Humphrey. 1986. A fresh look at genealogical bewilderment. *British Journal of Medical Psychology* 59:133–40.

Levy-Shiff, R., E. Vakil, L. Dimitrovsky, M. Abramovitz, N. Shahar, D. Hareven, S. Gross, M. Lerman, I. Levy, L. Sirota, and B. Fish. 1998. Medical, cognitive, emotional, and behavioral outcomes in school-age children conceived by in-vitro fertilization. *Journal of Clinical Child Psychology* 27:320–29.

Lewin, T. 2001. In genetic testing for paternity, law often lags behind science. *New York Times*, 11 March.

McLanahan, S., and G. Sandefur. 1994. *Growing Up with a Single Parent: What Hurts, What Helps.* Cambridge: Harvard University Press.

Melanson, Y. 1999. *Looking for Lost Bird.* New York: Avon Books.

Mendenhall, T. J., H. D. Grotevant, and R. G. McRoy. 1996. Adoptive couples: Communication and changes made in openness levels. *Family Relations* 45:223–29.

Parke, R. D., and P. N. Stearns. 1993. Fathers and child rearing. In *Children in Time and Place: Developmental and Historical Insights*, ed. G. H. Elder, J. Modell, and R. D. Parke, 147–70. Cambridge: Cambridge University Press.

Paternity of Cheryl. 2001. 746 N.E.2d 488 (Mass.).

Patterson, C. J., S. Hurt, and C. D. Mason. 1998. Families of the lesbian baby boom: Children's contact with grandparents and other adults. *American Journal of Orthopsychiatry* 68:390–99.

Quittner, A. L., L. C. Opipari, M. J. Regoli, J. Jacobsen, and H. Eigen. 1992. The impact of caregiving and role strain on family life: Comparisons between mothers of children with cystic fibrosis and matched controls. *Rehabilitation Psychology* 37:289–304.

Reid, M., S. L. Ramey, and M. Burchinal. 1990. Dialogues with children about their families. *New Directions for Child Development* 48:5–27.

Rohner, R. P. 1998. Father love and child development: History and current evidence. *Current Directions in Psychological Science* 7:157–61.

Rumball, A., and V. Adair. 1999. Telling the story: Parents' scripts for donor offspring. *Human Reproduction* 14:1392–99.

Snarey, J. 1993. *How Fathers Care for the Next Generation.* Cambridge: Harvard University Press.

Snarey, J., L. Son, V. S. Kuehne, S. Hauser, and G. Vaillant. 1987. The role of parenting in men's psychosocial development: A longitudinal study of early adulthood infertility and midlife generativity. *Developmental Psychology* 23:593–603.

Tamis-LeMonda, C. S., and N. Cabrera. 1999. Perspectives on father involvement: Research and policy. *Society for Research in Child Development Social Policy Report* 13:1–26.

Weiss, A., D. Scott-Jones, J. Ventrone, D. Vo, and M. Latimer-Sport. 2004. Current views on creating families: Perceptions of adoption and assisted reproduction. Paper presented at the biennial meeting of the Society for Research on Adolescence, Baltimore.

Wise v. Fryar. 2002. 49 S.W.3d 450 (Tex. Ct. App. 2001), *cert. denied,* 534 U.S. 1079.

Woodson, B. W. 2001. *A President in the Family: Thomas Jefferson, Sally Hemings, and Thomas Woodson.* Westport, CT: Praeger.

CHAPTER FIVE

Family Therapists and Parentage Testing

Dan Wulff, Ph.D.

Because all families are unique, the efforts of family therapists to characterize them in general categories undermine our ability to understand and assist them. Although family therapists have knowledge about families gained through experience and education, we need to approach each family with openness and receptiveness so that we can engender cooperative and durable working relationships. It is important to understand and appreciate how every family is structured to meet its needs and aspirations, sometimes in very different ways from other families. A family's reaction(s) to genetic parentage testing can be ascertained only through direct and perhaps prolonged inter-action with that family within a relationship of trust. All general understandings of families and their patterns of behavior ought to be held "lightly," creating a preparedness for the new, the novel, and the particular.

Paternity determinations are sought for a variety of reasons, only some of which are based on a concern for the well-being of the children. Clear and shared definitions of what constitutes a father, mother, child, and grandparent are less assured now than they once were. To be sure, some groups in society maintain firm definitions of these roles, but the proliferation of alternative family forms and relationships over the past thirty years has marked a decided trend toward a variability and uncertainty of definition. The expansion of family forms and relationships has come about gradually—a new marital arrangement here, a parenting adjustment there. Each adaptation has been met with some surprise and angst among those immediately affected, but most families and therapists eventually found a way of altering rigid standards and expectations. New language came along to describe these evolving variations. Whereas we once spoke of a "parent," we now can specify a *custodial* parent, a *genetic* or *biological* parent, or a *social* parent. These modifiers stretch the original definition to include categories that were once nonexistent or, at least, unacknowledged.

So we find ourselves in American society today amidst a great number of family variations—so numerous as to be more common than traditional normative forms. Recently, my wife's daughter (my stepdaughter) had a baby, and I began wondering about how my relationship with that child would or should develop. Will my role as a stepgrandfather differ from that of the biological grandfather? I posed this question to a graduate class in family therapy that I was teaching. Many students told stories about significant grandparent relationships that varied greatly in terms of the persons they referred to as grandparents—their biological connectedness seemed of less importance than the nature of their face-to-face interactions. The upshot of this discussion was that family roles are highly variable, and particular patterns of understanding and valuing grandparenting are idiosyncratic.

When family therapists work with families today, they must be alert to unique family structures and patterns and be ready to relate to each family with a healthy appreciation of that family's way(s) of construing or configuring family roles. This does not mean that we must accept or validate all family forms just because they exist. Nevertheless, any effort to assist or transform a family must first take stock of how the family members see themselves in relation to one another. This would apply to any professional helper, whether therapist, lawyer, physician, social worker, teacher, or minister. In this chapter I examine these ideas in relation to working with families in which parentage is at issue, highlighting specific ways to respect individual family variations.

Family as a System

In the field of psychotherapy, family therapy is the discipline that has the family as its focus. Other branches of therapy may take stock of the role and influence of family in the lives of their clients/patients as a way to better understand them, but approaching the family constellation as the principal locus of interest is the domain of the family therapist.

The family therapist attends to the family *as a unit* while considering individuals as *fragments* of the family. Individuals are viewed as subsystems that, although integral actors within the family system, cannot represent the overall functioning of the system. Individual problematic behaviors are considered to be signals of a family's distress rather than representative of autonomous individual acts or pathologies. Family therapy traces its development in the United States to the early 1950s, coalescing around a rather countercultural notion at the time (and, to a certain extent, still today) that individuals' behaviors could be more readily understood and approached by attending to their most immediate social context—their family.

The issue of parentage testing could appear in family therapy if the family (or some members) believed that confirming biological relatedness through scientific testing would be in some way helpful to their family and their relationships. A family therapist would consider this both as a substantive, material issue worthy of resolution and as reflective of the family's ongoing patterns of interaction with one another. How the family perceives this issue and what it hopes the testing will provide are critical information for the family therapist. For example, the testing may be used as a way to influence a family member to do something (or to stop doing something) more than as an effort to establish fact through a scientific process. More than any other purpose, finding out who the biological father is may serve the economic interests of family members.

Another way of saying this is that parentage testing could be appropriated by a family or a family member for a purpose other than what the procedure is designed to provide. In fact, for a family therapist, the context of the decision to pursue (or not pursue) parentage testing reveals as much as, if not more than, the test itself. It foreshadows the implications of the testing and allows us to understand the consequences for the family—not in terms of whether paternity is confirmed or disconfirmed, but rather in terms of what degree of credibility any test or externally generated evaluation will have for the collective perspective of the family or any of its members.

Who Comprises a Family?

Family membership itself is a variable notion, subject to very different traditions. "In some cultures, such as African American, West Indian, and Latino, close friends, neighbors, godparents, and members of the 'church family' may also be considered members of the family" (Boyd-Franklin and Bry 2000, 3). Even within a single family (however defined), various situations or decisions may enlist different people as members of the family at different times and

places. Given that family configurations often can include nonbiologically related members, there are numerous variables surrounding paternity testing.

A 2002 California Supreme Court decision said that "biology does not necessarily establish the only claim to parenthood and that, in some cases, parenthood can also be achieved through love and responsible conduct" (Janofsky,
in *In re Raphael P.* 2002). New terms such as *social father* are often invoked to
capture the role of a person who performs the functions of a father, even
though he is not the biological father. There are some who advocate dropping
the *social* designation in favor of giving the title *father* to a person who "acts
like a father." Changing *father* from a biological term to a behavioral one is
happening in practice in many cases, but legal and societal definitions still
maintain the preference for the biological definition. As more terms are used
that make finer distinctions to describe the roles or behaviors of fathers, the
dimensions of the social discourse surrounding fathers and their roles within
families continue to expand.

In discussions of family life and the roles of fathers, an "ideal" arrangement is often invoked, but, in practice, we see many adaptations of this ideal.
What we actually do in our families is more often a function of what is feasible and reasonable for us rather than of living up to an idealistic universal
image. For example, a child may have multiple sets of parents. With divorce
and remarriage, children may find themselves with two sets of parents—two
biological parents and two stepparents. The connections with the stepparents may include significant amounts of time spent at key developmental
points in the child's life.

Cultural Influences on Families

How one sees culture as an operative factor in the life of individual families drives one's effort to be responsive to those influences (Dean 2001). Some
notions of culture approach different groups "as sharing some essential characteristics that define them" (625). A family therapist approaching culture in
this way would seek to acquire knowledge about these defining characteristics. Cultures may be said to vary in the following areas of family life:

- Cultural attitudes, values, and traditions toward marriage and divorce;
- Spousal and gender roles and distribution of power in a marriage;
- Attitudes, customs, and learned behaviors regarding the discipline of children;

- Parent-child alignments and parent-child sleeping customs;
- Cultural attitudes and learned behavior about the expression of emotions;
- The self-esteem of a minority group member relative to the dominant society; and
- Concepts of time (Vasquez 1999, 159–60).

The term *cultural influence* often evokes images of ethnic or racial characteristics or traditions. Coming to understand a person or family as a simple replica of an ethnic or racial group drastically oversimplifies those so labeled. A plethora of external or cultural factors shape us throughout our lives, some of which are connected to our ethnic heritage or racial affiliation. But many such influences are not ethnic or racial—religious background, geographic region, rural/urban experiences, sexual orientation, educational/professional allegiances, socioeconomic status, or gender influences. It is also highly probable that these influences will not be static over the life course.

Dean (2001) suggests that gathering knowledge of cultures is, in itself, insufficient to successful work in cross-cultural contexts. She advocates that "we distrust the experience of 'competence' and replace it with a state of mind in which we are interested, and open but always tentative about what we understand" (629). When involved in an effort to predict or anticipate aspects of a family's life or beliefs, "it's important to remember that most families will gladly educate the therapist who shows genuine interest in their values and customs. An ability to be curious and respectful will get therapists further than an encyclopedic knowledge of what to expect from different kinds of families" (Nichols and Schwartz 2001, 322).

Beyond general group characteristics or demographics, we all exhibit a uniqueness not captured by expectations generated from our membership in these groupings. We may behave "out of character" at times, judged as unpredictable from our usual patterns of behavior. Each person is an amalgam of many affiliations, not just one. And these influences are in a fluid state of changing and incorporating new influences, so to characterize individuals or families along cultural lines is more complex than simply associating them with their racial or ethnic group.

Indeed, each family may be construed to be operating within a different set of understandings and preferences—of possessing its own "culture" (DiNicola 1997). In fact, judging each family as a unique culture may protect us from stereotyping or reifying persons or groups and help keep us in an inquisitive mode of "not-knowing" (Anderson and Goolishian 1992) and continuously learning. Such a posture will, in large measure, ensure that we approach clients in respectful ways that acknowledge their uniqueness a priori, itself a valuing approach.

Parentage testing is an issue that touches many belief systems held by families. Many specific beliefs or customs can be affected in complex ways, some negatively and some positively, and some positively and negatively simultaneously. Often, the attitudes toward testing vary according to whether such tests substantiate what the family expects or desires. At other times, the idea of an external "authority" asserting its opinion into a family situation is itself onerous, regardless of the findings.

Cultural difference can also be approached from a sociopolitical perspective that highlights "the way that group is treated within the larger culture" (Dean 2001, 626). Many ethnic minority families and communities have continuing relationships with legal entities or other institutions characterized by racism and prejudice (Boyd-Franklin 1989). "An important consequence of the experience of African American families with the history of racism and discrimination in the United States is the development of 'healthy cultural suspicion'" (Boyd-Franklin and Bry 2000, 13). A combination of suspiciousness and uncooperativeness may be a large player in how disenfranchised families relate to legal, medical, or educational institutions. A legal action (such as parentage testing) could be regarded as suspect by persons who have suffered at the hands of legal judgments. "Multigenerational experiences with racism, rejection, and the intrusion of agencies perpetuated by the welfare system have helped to create in many African American families a view that family dynamics are 'nobody's business but our own.' Members protect such families from intrusion by being secretive and sometimes unresponsive to outside interventions" (Boyd-Franklin and Bry 2000, 13). So, even potentially beneficial outcomes from parentage testing may be ignored because of a historical tradition of being suspicious of governmental or legal bodies.

Meanings for Clients

Meanings held by clients carry more weight than historical facts. The category of "married or not married" may hold various meanings or values— not a singular one. "Conflict in marriage" may be construed as a problem or as typical behavior, depending on the family. If we depend on categories of behavior to be consistent and essentialistic, we will often miss the significant meanings ascribed by those exhibiting these behaviors.

Even though universal definitions and meanings for fatherhood are not possible, the prevalence of biological interests and the influential place of lineage are undeniable. But simply to say that biology is the key element is to erroneously downplay the roles of other factors.

Results of scientific tests to discover paternity may be set aside by families or family members who choose to believe something contrary. Several types of logic may exist—*legal* logic, predicated on laws, statutes, and legal precedents, or *family logic,* based on customary ways in which a family has understood things. In the legal arena, legal logic prevails; in the family life arena, family logic prevails. This is not to say that there is no overlap of these two types of logic, but the world can be construed very differently when viewing situations from one point of view or the other. If a family has an investment in a specific outcome in a paternity issue, it has numerous ways to maintain its view, even in the face of contrary scientific evidence. The family can assert that those in charge of the testing behaved in negligent or biased ways. It can even dismiss science altogether. The desire to claim a child or to deny a relationship to a child for familial reasons can trump (at least in the mind of those so inclined) scientific or legal results. Parties contesting the parentage of a child can see their positions as a battle of wills or as a measure of the level of commitment. Even though legal or scientific judgments may carry the day, the ramifications of a split between a family's view and the legal system's decision may be significant for decades in the lives of those so involved, including the lives of children.

The legal logic position valorizes concepts such as "in the best interests of the child." In families, the best interests of the child(ren) are factored into "other" best interests—those of the other members of the family. Parceling best interests as competing concepts within a family oversimplifies the task of providing for multiple individuals within a social unit and within a larger community. Because of abuses of children and their lack of power within families, the legal system has sought to address the needs of children through legal protections and interpretations. In the arena of paternity testing, issues of whose best interests are being served are, at best, muddied, and the legal system is hard pressed to locate a determination that clearly and unequivocally serves the best interests of the child in the broadest sense of the term.

As in most issues that affect families, competing and concurrent interests are involved. When one is deliberating and deciding how to handle a specific issue, the interests of each family member, of subgroups, and of society at large are all implicated. Family therapists and their clients need to have a mutual adjustment of interests rather than a singular prevailing concern.

Parentage testing is often used as a tool for certain parental interests to achieve their desired outcomes, and claiming the best-interests-of-the-child doctrine may be a tactic to gain what the parent feels is in his or her own best interest. Contentious family situations or relationships frequently provide the setting in which certain individuals within a family can use parentage-testing procedures to further their individual agendas. Rather than agreeing to use parentage testing as a vehicle to settle family disputes, families may use such testing to stimulate or further family discord—parentage testing thus becomes a pawn in a more encompassing chess game. When parents and their representatives argue for what is in the best interests of their child, how do family therapists separate that issue from what is in the best interests of the parent? From what standpoint can anyone speak for the best interests of the child? Who will accurately represent the best interests of the child in question? Clearly, paternity testing may be pursued as a means to advance the economic interests of one or both of the parents.

Respectful Questions

The variety of family forms, customs, processes, and beliefs can have the benefit of loosening our ethnocentric beliefs that suggest our personal views are essentially correct. Spanning the various possibilities of how families, parents, and children relate to one other gives us a range of thinking that could allow us to receive other views (distinct from our own) with a grace and respect (verbally and nonverbally) that might not otherwise be present.

Madsen (1999) uses the phrase "cultural curiosity" to "refer to a continual attempt to actively elicit a client's particular meaning rather than assume we already know it or that it is the same as ours" (158). The answer to this challenge may be to develop the ability to ask open-ended, curiosity-motivated questions of our clients. The goal leads us to understand another cultural entity (family), inclusive of how they see themselves. "A therapeutic conversation is no more than a slowly evolving and detailed, concrete, individual life story stimulated by the therapist's position of not-knowing and the therapist's curiosity to learn" (Anderson and Goolishian 1992, 38). The professional who is interested in families can ask questions that may extend the family's own understanding of itself. Indeed, such questioning requires a sense of safety in the relationship with the questioner. Relationships characterized by intimidation, fear, or dread do not present the possibility for such generative conversations. To the extent that parentage testing is seen as a legal action, clients may be wary, and that impediment to a "safe" relationship would need to be addressed.

Significantly open-ended questions allow families to present their views, usually in ways unanticipated by the questioner. These questions, by their structure, convey to families a respect for their views—a key component of any working relationship with a family. The following is a sample of questions that could be used to discern how a family (or family member) feels about identity testing.

What do children mean to your family? This invites stories about how children are viewed within the family unit—the roles they play in the family's understanding of itself, the feelings associated with children, relationships between parents and children, and the importance of the family name.

What is your view about parentage testing? This invites the respondents to describe what they know about the procedure, along with their respect (or lack thereof) for such methods. This may lead family members to ask questions about such tests to fill in the gaps in their knowledge.

How might you react to the various possible outcomes of a parentage test? This future-oriented question asks them to consider the various outcomes and to anticipate their feelings attached to each potential result. This would allow the respondents to comment on the credibility of such tests in the context of their family.

What might be the most difficult aspect(s) of a parentage test for your family? This invites the family members to locate where the stresses would be: in deciding whether to proceed with the testing? In facing the outcomes? In the anger or sadness that might be forthcoming?

Who is likely to have the toughest time with such a test? Who might benefit the most? How might this affect the child? This invites speculation about those family members who are most invested in the outcomes, those whose emotional reactions may be most charged.

What is the likelihood that a parentage test would resolve the issues within the families involved? This asks for an opinion about whether this test would solve whatever the test was intended to solve or if other things would be needed. It allows the family to express doubts about the test.

Who should be involved in making the decision about whether to undergo this test? The family should be invited to discuss the process of deciding whether this test should be conducted as well as any other parameters of its administration.

What would be the best way to resolve this issue? Can everyone involved be satisfied? If not, what should be done? This question invites the respondents to offer their opinions about what would be most helpful in this situation. They may reaffirm or reject the parentage test. If the respondents' viewpoints can be utilized, their input can be a problem-solving opportunity.

These questions, asked of the families involved in the parentage dispute, can improve the degree of buy-in of all parties, a situation superior to one in which opposition becomes entrenched. The questions must be asked honestly and asked of all parties. And, to the extent possible, information received that can be acted on should be. If the questions seem perfunctory or administrative only, the family members will not see the questions as serving them in any way—only as some paperwork requirement or, worse yet, an attempt to build a case that one day may be used against them.

In approaching the issue of parentage testing and its effects on families, one might take a strict legal approach that attempts to place the issue into clear, carefully defined categories from which decisions can be predictably achieved. Or one could maintain a multifaceted and complex appreciation of parentage testing that privileges each family's struggles in ways that cannot be predicted. The choice may be characterized as between a simple, flawed solution versus a nuanced, cumbersome solution. These decisions may come down to a choice based on the ultimate purposes of the decision makers. The needs of society to have laws that order and regularize family life and decisions about family membership are placed alongside the needs of families to be free to conduct their family life and the accompanying decisions therein according to the customs and patterns each family has developed. How do we accommodate these often competing sets of legitimate needs?

Laws support the maintenance of an ordered or patterned form of interaction. In that sense, they become regulating and serve to perpetuate existing behaviors. While statutes maintain order and consistency, new societal discourse around key organizing features of the community can push the limits of our system to include more variations in behavior. Cultural artifacts (e.g., movies, music, celebrities, critical events) can move our understandings and appreciations into arenas not covered by current behavior and organization. The debates surrounding parentage testing can stimulate social dialogue about what makes a family, what makes a parent, and what makes a father. This issue could be instrumental in transforming what constitutes a family or in maintaining our current conceptualizations.

The more one works with families involved with parentage testing, the more one comes to know the differing issues and reactions of families to the experience. The wise family therapist will translate those understandings into an appreciative stance toward families and the varieties and similarities of their responses, confident in what he or she has witnessed and ever prepared to see something new.

BIBLIOGRAPHY

Anderson, H., and H. Goolishian. 1992. The client is the expert: A not-knowing approach to therapy. In *Therapy as Social Construction,* ed. S. McNamee and K. J. Gergen, 25–39. London: Sage.

Boyd-Franklin, N. 1989. *Black Families in Therapy: A Multisystems Approach.* New York: Guilford Press.

Boyd-Franklin, N., and B. H. Bry. 2000. *Reaching Out in Family Therapy: Home-Based, School, and Community Interventions.* New York: Guilford Press.

Dean, R. G. 2001. The myth of cross-cultural competence. *Families in Society: The Journal of Contemporary Human Services* 8:623–30.

DiNicola, V. 1997. *A Stranger in the Family: Culture, Families, and Therapy.* New York: W. W. Norton.

In re Raphael P. 2002. 118 Cal. Rptr. 2d 610 (Cal. Ct. App.).

Madsen, W. C. 1999. *Collaborative Therapy with Multi-Stressed Families: From Old Problems to New Futures.* New York: Guilford Press.

Nichols, M. P., and R. C. Schwartz. 2001. *Family Therapy: Concepts and Methods,* 5th ed. Boston: Allyn and Bacon.

Vasquez, R. 1999. Cultural issues in evaluations. In *Complex Issues in Child Custody Evaluations,* ed. P. M. Stahl, 153–68. Thousand Oaks, CA: Sage.

CHAPTER SIX

From Genes, Marriage, and Money to Nurture

Redefining Fatherhood

Nancy E. Dowd, J.D., Ph.D.

We are poised at the threshold of establishing genetic fatherhood for all children. This technological development and capability intersects with social and political changes in our definition of fatherhood that have also affected its legal definition. Largely in the name of gender equality and to some extent in the name of children's rights, we have moved from a legal definition of fatherhood linked to marriage toward a legal definition of fatherhood linked to genes. Although historically fatherhood existed almost exclusively within marriage, we have moved to include nonmarital fathers within our legal definitions primarily to obtain monetary support for children. Currently, fatherhood is defined primarily in economic terms. At the same time, notions of gender equity have removed formal barriers to the custody and nurture of children by their fathers, although child care disproportionately remains in the mother's hands (Fitzgerald 1994). This acknowledgment of men's ability to nurture and parent, however, has remained far secondary to defining men's role as purely economic, within the classic paradigm of the breadwinner.

DNA technology has the capability to solidify this movement from marriage to genetic definitions of parenting and to define fathering as a status that generates the duty of economic support. DNA technology could also be the basis for establishing genetic identification for all children for the purpose of obtaining economic support from their genetic fathers. No longer would we have "deadbeat dads," because genetic fatherhood would be established and better collection mechanisms would ensure greater economic support for children. Similarly, we would no longer have "duped dads," men who thought their children were "theirs," subsequently discover they have no genetic connection, but nevertheless retain legal obligations linked to the birth of those children during marriage and the operation of legal rules that presume fatherhood. DNA technology can be the basis to argue for an end to the marital presumption, whereby the children of a marriage are presumed to be the biological children of the married couple (*Michael H. v. Gerald D.* 1989). Genetic ties would link fathers to children and would be the basis of legal obligation and, by implication, legal rights.

Genes should not define fatherhood. This is wrong for men and wrong for children. Genes define identity, but that link should be separated from the obligations and rights of parenthood. By *identity,* I mean genes provide critical information about parentage that might be necessary for medical decisions or for knowing and identifying with racial or ethnic heritage. Specifically, I argue that fatherhood should be defined by *doing* (action) instead of *being* (status), with the critical component being the acts of nurturing. Throughout this discussion of fatherhood, genetic ties, and the policy implications of defining fatherhood around nurture when genetic ties can be established for all children, it is critical to remain cognizant of the diversity of fathers and the fluidity of fatherhood. Not all fathers are alike, and fatherhood is not a fixed state.

Defining Fatherhood as Nurture

When defining fatherhood with respect to legal rights and responsibilities, one is tempted to think formally in terms of status. If we define fatherhood by marriage or by genetic connection, it is relatively simple to identify who is a father. Similarly, it also becomes simple to identify who has responsibility, especially financial responsibility, for children. Although financial responsibility serves our social, adult needs, what matters most to children is emotional relationships and caregiving.

My redefinition of fatherhood centers fathering on nurture. This definition moves away from the marital model of traditional fatherhood and the bioeconomic model of recent legal reforms toward affirmative means to support men's nurture of children and their interconnections with mothers and other caretakers. It is a serious and radical change, because it cannot be achieved without confronting the economic support of children and implementing true egalitarian, cooperative, mutual support models of parenting. Accomplishing these goals for all children, not just privileged ones, is an enormous task. Economic policy is foremost. Limited or no economic support means class-limited fatherhood. Just as important as economic policy, however, is cultural policy. We must challenge entrenched concepts of masculinity and fatherhood (Burgess 1997). Redefining fatherhood requires redefining what it means to be a man.

I would define fatherhood around nurture, not around genetics or economic responsibilities. Fatherhood as nurture means fatherhood as function, not as status. Social fatherhood is the practice of nurture, either alone or in combination with other caretakers, as the sole or primary parent, or contributing as closely as possible to an equal amount of caregiving in partnership with the other primary parent or parents. In essence, it is nonexclusive, cooperative parenting.

Nurture is a rich concept, and by it I mean the psychological, physical, intellectual, and spiritual care and support of children. It must be seen in the context of development and thus is fluid, not fixed, in accord with children's needs. It is both qualitative and quantitative. Qualitatively, the focus of nurture is on children's well-being and the well-being of other caretakers, and this means child care is interconnected with other household work (Ehrensaft 1987). It is also linked to the interconnection of family work and wage work and the harmonization of fatherhood with motherhood (Coltrane and Valdez 1993). Quantitatively, it means shared responsibility, as close to fifty-fifty sharing as possible, but no less than sixty-forty, or otherwise proportionate to the presence of other caregivers. It is not secondary parenting; it is coequal parenting.

The full support of nurture means facing and resolving gender challenges to men's identification with caregiving. One gender challenge is the very definition of masculinity in anticare, antinurture terms, linked to the promotion of homophobia in the definition of masculinity (Epstein 1997). Caring is viewed as not manly and is marked in a way that makes care a conflict-ridden action for many men. Another significant gender challenge to supporting men's nurture is resolving tensions between fathers and mothers. These tensions block egalitarian parenthood and explode in the persistence of domestic violence.

Defining fatherhood around nurture must also include all fathers, for the benefit of all children. There are also race and class challenges in redefining fatherhood. Without an economic strategy, any redefinition of fatherhood will be confounded by the economic necessities of families and the gendered structure of the workplace. Without a cultural strategy, any redefinition of fatherhood will be formal rather than meaningful in the lives of children and men.

Implications of Fatherhood Defined around Nurture

A redefinition of fatherhood around nurture would lead not only to changes in existing legal structures but also, more significantly, to affirmative restructuring to achieve the goal of better nurture of children. The changes that would be triggered in existing structures and doctrines of family law can be summarized as completing the dismantling of patriarchal fatherhood. Under the common law, family was defined in patriarchal terms, with the man as the head of the household, his wife as a gender-defined, unequal partner, and children as the servants of the father as master. Although much of patriarchal fatherhood has disappeared under the emergence of egalitarian family norms, vestiges of patriarchy remain. One of these vestiges is the concept of illegitimacy. A second significant vestige is the link between the payment of money and entitlement to a social relationship that is present in practice, even if not in formal rules. These practices manifest in the custody, visitation, and child support framework within which divorced and nonmarital fathers function.

Affirmative restructuring necessary to accomplish redefined fatherhood is much more extensive and includes economic, cultural, and educational reforms. Economic restructuring must ensure sufficient economic child support so that fathers can nurture their children, rather than being confined to breadwinning as a result of gendered economic structures in the workplace. More broadly, work-family conflicts must be eliminated or significantly reduced. Culturally, fatherhood education is essential to reorient male norms and teach the skills and norms of redefined fatherhood (Dowd 2000). That reorientation can be especially effective at childbirth and divorce, two places where the state already is significantly involved in the family and where men have demonstrated strong interest in and commitment to fathering. Educational programs must teach nurture and confront cultural barriers with gender-specific, gender-relevant strategies.

It is essential to emphasize how critical economic policy is to the success of male nurture of children. The rate of child poverty in the United States, measured under the conservative federal definition of poverty, has ranged in the past decade between one in five and one in six children (Li and Bennet 1996).

At least some of that high poverty rate is attributable to the lack of paternal economic support of children who live in single-parent households. The possibilities for changing children's poverty include ensuring support payment under the existing system, providing backup support under the existing system, and supplementing that support when it is inadequate. A more serious effort to deal with child poverty would provide family support to all children sufficient to cover their basic needs beyond the current definition of poverty. However, such economic policies, whether limited or more radical, must be combined with increased efforts to eliminate gender- and race-based employment discrimination as well as implementing work and family policies that permit parents to parent children while engaging in wage work. Without such comprehensive economic policy making, men will be pushed by the gendered and racialized employment sector to engage in wage work over nurturing work. Therefore, economic necessity will undermine the needs of children for nurture from their fathers. Moreover, for some children, even two full-time working parents will not lift them out of poverty.

Implications of Redefining Fatherhood for Genetic Ties

It is tempting to use genetic ties to define fatherhood as a way to ensure children's welfare by scientifically identifying their fathers, but this is a false and limited solution to children's needs, as Bartholet indicates (chapter 8). Genes should not be the foundation on which legal fatherhood is established.

This does not mean that genes have no place in redefined fatherhood. Genes are a connection that we presume to be, and would support, as embedded within the relational connection to the mother and the child that generates a connection of care, which is the basis of redefined fatherhood. In other words, we would assume that in many if not most cases, nurture would coexist with genetic ties. Genetic ties are not, however, ownership rights that create rights of access.

Genetic ties create identity rights. Children have a right to know their genetic identity, most strongly for medical reasons, but also to value cultural pluralism and social identity. This would support a system of universal genetic identification and access to nonidentifying genetic information (Kaplan 2000). Genetic identification would disconnect identity from marriage and from the historic notion of "legitimacy" (Dowd 2000). All children would be "legitimate," based on their humanity, not on patriarchal claims. Alternatively, the very notion of legitimacy would disappear (*Michael H. v. Gerald D.* 1989). A child would be recognized individually, with genetic ties as part of his or her identity, and the child's parents would be identified by nurture and by action rather than by status.

In addition to rejecting the concept of legitimacy/illegitimacy, one could also make an argument for elimination of the marital presumption as we know it. The marital presumption functions to establish legitimacy and legal parenthood by assuming that any child born within a marriage is the child of the married couple (Cal. Fam. Code § 7540 [West 2003]). Universal genetic identification, rather than elective genetic identification, would squarely contradict the marital presumption. Nevertheless, if fatherhood is defined by action rather than by status, the legal father might be identified in one of two ways. First, the husband is always the legal father, under a theory of marriage that views the birth of children as a shared responsibility, regardless of genetic ties. What I am suggesting here is a truly egalitarian marriage, defined as shared parenting with respect to children (Fineman 1995). Alternatively, the actions of the potential father would be evaluated to establish legal fatherhood, defined by acts of nurture. Under the first approach, the functional consequence would be only slightly different from the operation of the marital presumption today, but our conceptions and rationalizations as well as the basis for imposing obligations would be different. Under the second approach, the outcome might be quite different from the current operation of the presumption, because either the husband or the genetic father, or both, could be a nurturing, social father. Under either approach, children are connected to parents not because of genetic imprint but because of intentional, ongoing caretaking. The process of adoption best exemplifies this model.

A second consequence of linking genes to identity but not to parental status is that economic responsibility and rights to social parenthood should not be linked (Josephson 1997; Czapanskiy 1991; Knitzer et al. 1997). In its most radical form, what I am proposing is that genetic fatherhood should not create economic responsibility that creates social or relational rights. In a less radical form, genetic fatherhood would generate economic responsibility but not relational rights; relational rights would be dependent on satisfying a definition of nurturing fatherhood. Economic support of children is critical to their well-being and must be a universal norm, irrespective of family form or the presence or absence of parents. Even if all fathers were identified and all child support as currently structured were paid, we would not eliminate a sub-

stantial proportion of child poverty. So we must implement policies that support children while also bearing in mind that children's core needs are not purely economic (Wambaugh 1999).

Linking social rights to economic responsibilities reinforces the notion of children as property, a classic hallmark of rejected patriarchal norms (Anderlik and Rothstein 2002). It also reinforces the role of fathers as breadwinners rather than nurturers, or defines nurture purely in economic terms when men are doing the nurturing. Any comprehensive effort to support children economically that includes the goal of supporting men's nurturing must reward and support noneconomic nurture and care.

Another corollary of this disconnection between dollars and parental rights is the support of parenting, particularly the support of nurturing fathers, a phenomenon that has largely been devalued and rendered invisible. One way in which this might be accomplished is through the elimination of joint *legal* custody, whereby fathers, whether occasional, joint, or coequal parents, are given power over decision making with respect to their children. At the same time, joint *physical* custody, whereby the care of children is presumptively equally shared, would be the norm for redefined fathers (Maxwell 1998; Fabricius and Braver 2003). The norm, instead of the exception, would be an expectation of fifty-fifty parenting. But most critically, work and family support must increase to ensure that the commitment to nurture can be realized without jeopardizing wage work.

Rather than using genetic ties to identify fathers, we should focus on supporting all fathers who nurture children. Genetic ties may create a false sense of fairness and equality, because every father should be a responsible father. But ignoring the differences in fathers' capabilities means allowing children to be treated differently based on their luck, or lack of it. It is critical, then, that fatherhood policy look at fathers at the margins and place them in the center of new policy directions. In this instance, "fathers at the margins" means those fathers who are nurturing at the margin from the standpoint of the central breadwinner/secondary parent model. It could also mean looking at men marginalized by race and class and ensuring that they can be a part of any new redefinition of fatherhood. Margins operate in several ways. Class and race margins make it more difficult for poor fathers and fathers of color to nurture. Black fathers must be viewed within the context of their status as black males. "They experience higher rates of unemployment, poverty, morbidity, and imprisonment and have shorter life expectancy, less access to health care, and less education than their white counterparts" (Cochran 1997, 342). Failing to take account of those differences perpetuates family inequalities that have significant implications for children's opportunities in life.

A different kind of marginalization is the variation in the kinds of fathers that engage in nurture and the societal support given to assist them in that task. Nonmarital fathers, stepfathers, and teen fathers are clearly identifiable as less visible, less supported, and less valued in social and cultural terms, although their care is often critical to children. Adoptive fathers and gay fathers are two other subsets of fathers that are rarely thought of when constructing social policy. The fathers at the margins have needs, but they also provide valuable lessons about fatherhood (Dowd 2000). We can better support them and the children they nurture, but we can also learn by observing how they have cared for their children despite the barriers and what different models contributed to their children's general welfare.

Evaluating Redefined Fatherhood

How radical a change would it be to redefine fatherhood around nurture? One way to analyze these issues is by referencing our current notions of fatherhood. This is the context in which most men become genetic fathers, usually by their twenties or thirties. However, many fathers never become nurturers during the span of their child's life. Of all fathers, a small number nurture their children in a way that we most strongly associate with mothers, either as primary or sole parents or, less commonly, in equal partnership with mothers. A larger number of fathers nurture as secondary parents. That is, they are back-up nurturers to mothers, but their nurture is distinctly secondary rather than coequal (Gerson 1993). A third pattern of fathers is those who are largely disengaged from their children, other than providing economic support. Finally, there are totally disengaged fathers, either because no connection was ever made or because they have drifted entirely out of their children's lives, both socially and economically. These patterns of fatherhood are strongly but not exclusively linked to whether men share a household with their children and to their relationship with the children's mothers. Men are more likely to nurture when they reside with their children, and they are more likely to nurture children when they have a good relationship with the children's mother.

Ironically, however, those men who share a household with their children's mother are not necessarily those who nurture the most; they are more likely to be secondary nurturers. The men who tend to nurture the most are primary parents (Dowd 2000).

Men's fathering is characteristically serial rather than linear. As men couple and uncouple with women, their nurturing tends to follow their adult relationships. Thus it is not uncommon that a man might father two sets of children, although not at the same time, and thus his relationship with children is not constant. Women, by contrast, are more likely to sustain a prolonged relationship with their children (Dowd 2000).

Fathers' impact on the lives of their children is positive, especially because their presence usually brings more economic resources, which in turn have a powerful effect on children's well-being. Mere presence of a father figure in the home, however, is not sufficient, even if economic well-being increases. That is apparent in the pattern of children in blended families, suggesting that stepfathers function in a distinctly different way.

Most significantly, fathers do not parent qualitatively in a way that is distinctive or unique. Their presence in children's lives is important and profound, but not because of uniqueness or gender essentialism (Dowd 2000). Rather, nurture by multiple adults benefits children, and nurture by engaged parents is fundamentally the same, irrespective of gender.

This discussion leaves many questions. Should we work within the existing patterns of fatherhood or try to change them? Should fatherhood be supported exclusively or preferentially within marriage? How do we empower fathers without subjugating mothers? Should we envision fatherhood as a single-parent or dual-parent role? Can we support nurturing fatherhood while insisting on financial responsibility? Will we continue to see financial responsibility in individual and unequal terms? How do we incorporate the fluidity and multiplicity of family structures and changes over time?

My answers, in brief, to these questions are that we should work to enhance the patterns of nurture by removing the barriers to fathers' ability to nurture their children. Rather than trying to reorient men's household pattern, we can support their nurture of the children that they live with as well as support, if they choose, the nurture of children that no longer share their daily life. To prefer fatherhood within marriage, and thus return to the distinction between children within and outside marriage, defies demographic patterns but also, most significantly, stigmatizes and harms children because of adult choices over which children have no control.

Empowering fathers without reconstituting gender inequality requires that we not look at fatherhood in isolation or cast fathers' rights as independent of the need for positive interrelationship with mothers. In addition, if fatherhood is viewed under a shared, co-parenting model, as opposed to conceptualizing it as a primary parent model in which men equally serve as primary parents, this contributes to equal empowerment and relational balance but also requires resolving the puzzle of economic support of families and a re-orientation of work and family structures. It likely means public as well as private support of families, not limited to needs-based support.

Incorporating the fluidity of family forms and their changes over time means focusing on what fathers and families do, rather than what they look like. Our goal should be the long-term well-being of all children, which requires bringing the interests of those children with the greatest needs to the center of policy making. The policies that we need to adopt must be measured against the needs of those at the margins.

Conclusion

The tragedy of September 11, 2001, brought many things into focus. In the months that followed, the *New York Times* began to write unique obituaries about those who had died, stories that captured the essence of lives cut short, as many of those who died were quite young (New York Times 2002). It became apparent that young men were disproportionately killed in the 9/11 attacks, because a large percentage of business people in the World Trade Towers were young men. Many were fathers. Some were soon to become fathers. There were also fathers left among the survivors who could not easily be linked to the children they were left to nurture, or who were suddenly thrust into that role because of genetics or prior marital connections. It also became apparent, as support for families affected by 9/11 became a priority, that not all surviving fathers would meet common legal definitions (Dowd 2003). Not all were linked by marriage to the mothers, and some could not have married the partners whose children they nurtured. This tragedy was a window on how we live and love and care for others. Of the many lessons it has to teach us, surely one is that it is the active work of caring and loving rather than our passive, genetic makeup that matters the most.

BIBLIOGRAPHY

Abbott, J. D. 1999. Annual survey of Michigan law June 1, 1997–May 31, 1998. *Wayne Law Review* 45:973–1057.

Anderlik, M. R., and M. A. Rothstein. 2002. DNA-based identity testing and the future of the family: A research agenda. *American Journal of Law and Medicine* 28:215–32.

Blankenhorn, D. 1995. *Fatherless America: Confronting Our Most Urgent Social Problem.* New York: Basic Books.

Burgess, A. 1997. *Fatherhood Reclaimed: The Making of the Modern Father.* London: Vermillion.

Chambers, D. 1984. Rethinking the substantive rules for custody disputes in divorce. *Michigan Law Review* 83:477–569.

Cochran, D. L. 1997. African American fathers: A decade review of the literature. *Families in Society* 78:340–51.

Collier, R. 1995a. *Masculinity Law and the Family.* New York: Routledge.

———. 1995b. Waiting till father gets home: The reconstruction of fatherhood in family law. *Social and Legal Studies* 4:5–30.

Coltrane, S., and E. O. Valdez. 1993. Reluctant compliance: Work-family role allocation in dual-earner Chicano families. In *Men, Work and Families,* ed. J. C. Hood, 163–69. Newbury Park, CA: Sage.

Costello, C., and B. Kivimae. 1996. *The American Woman 1996–97: Where We Stand—Women and Work.* New York: W. W. Norton.

Czapanskiy, K. 1991. Volunteers and draftees: The struggle for parental equality. *UCLA Law Review* 38:1415–80.

Dolgin, J. L. 2001. Choice, tradition and the new genetics: The fragmentation of the ideology of family. *Connecticut Law Review* 32:523–66.

Dowd, N. E. 2000. *Redefining Fatherhood.* New York: New York University Press.

———. 2003. Symposium: Law, culture, and family: The transformative power of culture and the limits of the law. *Chicago-Kent Law Review* 78:785–806.

Ehrenreich, B. 1983. *The Hearts of Men: American Dreams and the Flight from Commitment.* New York: Anchor.

Ehrensaft, D. 1987. *Parenting Together: Men and Women Sharing the Care of Their Children.* New York: Free Press.

Epstein, D. 1997. Boys' own stories: Masculinities and sexualities in schools. *Gender and Education* 9:105–16.

Fabricius, W. V., and S. L. Braver. 2003. Non-child support expenditures on children by non-residential divorced fathers: Results of a study. In Separated and Unmarried Fathers and the Courts, special issue. *Family Court Review* 41:321–36.

Fineman, M. 1995. *The Neutered Mother, the Sexual Family, and Other Twentieth Century Tragedies.* New York: Routledge.

Finkler, K. 2001. The kin in the gene: Medicalization of family and kinship in American society. *Current Anthropology* 42:235–63.

Fitzgerald, W. 1994. Maturity, difference, and mystery: Children's perspectives and the law. *Arizona Law Review* 36:11–111.

Garfinkel, I., and P. Wong. 1990. Child support and public policy. In *Lone Parent Families: The Economic Challenge,* ed. E. Duskin. Paris: Organization for Economic Cooperation and Development.

Gerson, K. 1993. *No Man's Land: Men's Changing Commitments to Family and Work*. New York: Basic Books.

———. 1997. An institutional perspective on generative fathering: Creating social supports for parenting equality. In *Generative Fathering: Beyond Deficit Perspectives*, ed. A. J. Hawkins. Thousand Oaks, CA: Sage.

Hawkins, A. J., and D. C. Dollahite, eds. 1997. *Generative Fathering: Beyond Deficit Perspectives*. Thousand Oaks, CA: Sage.

In re J.W.T. 1994. 872 S.W.2d 189, 194 (Tex.).

Josephson, J. J. 1997. *Gender, Families and State: Child Support Policy in the United States*. Lanham, MD: Rowman and Littlefield.

Kaplan, D. S. 2000. Why truth is not a defense in paternity actions. *Texas Journal of Women and Law* 10:69–81.

Kimbrell, A. 1995. *The Masculine Mystique: The Politics of Masculinity*. New York: Ballantine Books.

Kimmel, M. S. 1988. *Changing Men: New Directions in Research on Men and Masculinity*. New York: Sage.

Knitzer, J., E. Brenner, S. Bernard, and V. Gadsen. 1997. *Map and Track: State Initiatives to Encourage Responsible Fatherhood*. New York: Columbia University School of Public Health, National Center for Children.

Li, J., and N. Bennet. 1996. *One in Four: America's Youngest Poor*. New York: National Council of Churches.

Maxwell, K. E. 1998. Preventative lawyering strategies to mitigate the detrimental effects of clients' divorces on their children. *Review Journal of the University of Puerto Rico* 67:137–64.

McEwen, J. A. 2000. Genetic information, ethics, and information relating to biological parenthood. In *Encyclopedia of Ethical, Legal, and Policy Issues in Biotechnology*, ed. T. H. Murray and M. J. Melhman, 356–63. Indianapolis: Wiley.

McNeely, C. 1998. Lagging behind the times: Parenthood, custody, and gender bias in the family court. *Florida State University Law Review* 25:891–956.

Michael H. v. Gerald D. 1989. 491 U.S. 110, 115, 117.

Nelkin, D., and S. Lindee. 1995. *The DNA Mystique: The Gene as a Cultural Icon*. New York: W. H. Freeman.

New York Times. 2002. *Portraits: 9/11/01: The Collected "Portraits of Grief" from the New York Times*. New York: The Times.

Parness, J. A. 1993. Designating male parents at birth. *University of Michigan Journal of Law Reform* 26:573–92.

Popenhoe, D. 1996. *Life without Father: Compelling New Evidence That Fatherhood and Marriage Are Indispensable for the Good of Children and Society*. New York: Free Press.

Robinson, B., and S. Parker. 2001. Who is daddy? A case for the Uniform Parentage Act. *Delaware Lawyer* 19:23–24.

Schoonmaker, S. V. 1997. Consequences and validity of family law provisions in the welfare reform act. *Journal of the American Academy of Matrimonial Lawyers* 14:3–72.

Shapiro, E. D., S. Reifler, and C. L. Psome. 1992–93. The DNA paternity test: Legislating the future paternity action. *Journal of Law and Health* 7:1–50.

Snarey, J. 1993. *How Fathers Care for the Next Generation: A Four Decade Study*. Cambridge: Harvard University Press.

Taylor, R. J., J. S. Jackson, and L. M. Chatters, eds. 1997. *Family Life in Black America.* Thousand Oaks, CA: Sage.

Wambaugh, C. L. 1999. Biology is important, but does not necessarily always constitute a family: A brief survey of the Uniform Adoption Act. *Akron Law Review* 32:791–832.

Weir, R. F., S. Lawrence, and E. Fales, eds. 1994. *Genes and Human Self Knowledge: Historical and Philosophical Reflections on Modern Genetics.* Iowa City: University of Iowa Press.

Woodhouse, B. B. 1993. Hatching the egg: A child-centered perspective on parents' rights. *Cardozo Law Review* 14:1747–1806.

Part II / Parentage in American Family Law

Trends and Recommendations

CHAPTER SEVEN

Duped Dads and Discarded Children

A Historical Perspective on DNA Testing in Child Custody Cases

Michael Grossberg, Ph.D.

In 1992, Gerald Miscovich filed suit in Pennsylvania in an attempt to avoid paying support for a son born to his wife, Elizabeth Miscovich, during their marriage. The boy was born in 1987, and the pair divorced in 1990. In 1992, Gerald had himself and the child genetically tested. The test excluded Gerald as the boy's biological father, making him, he charged, a duped dad. Within months he told the child the test results and terminated his relationship with the boy. He then filed suit to end his child support payments. Elizabeth tried to hold a third party responsible and sought a blood test to determine her son's paternity. The trial court refused to order blood testing or to admit the DNA evidence that Gerald had obtained. On appeal, Gerald argued that the courts should recognize DNA evidence of paternity. He asked the judges to reject the centuries-old common law rule that children born within a marriage are presumed to have been fathered by the husband. Doing so would also mean rejecting the traditional logic that, because paternity could never be proven without a doubt, excluding evidence of infidelity was the best way to protect children from the stigma of illegitimacy, men from the shame of cuckoldry, and society from marital disruption and child support. But, Gerald insisted, DNA testing had transformed the situation. Paternity could now be established with scientific certainty and thus the old policy should be cast aside in the interests of fairness and justice. Duped dads should, in other words, be given the legal right to discard other men's children.

Pennsylvania judges disagreed. In 1995, a state appellate court concluded that the presumption should continue and that Gerald had not offered evidence of the traditional grounds for rebutting it: proof of his sterility, impotence, or nonaccess to his wife. They did, however, acknowledge that the presumption might well be reexamined in the light of "advancements in technology." "We need not," the court explained, "blindly apply [the presumption], nor cling to timeworn principles to support the Commonwealth's goal of protecting the family" (*Miscovich v. Miscovich* 1997). However, the judges concluded that a case-by-case evaluation of the evidence should be used to assess claims like Gerald's. They then ruled that the evidence argued in favor of presuming his paternity of the boy.

> Here Gerald clearly had an established relationship with his son . . . He did not question it until after the relationship between him and his wife deteriorated. Although the family is not now intact . . . familial relationship existed at the time the child was born, and more significantly, a parent-child bond was formed. Despite Gerald's unilateral termination of this relationship and his decision to notify the child that he was not his father, we find that a considered application of the myriad factors involved to the facts of this case warrant a finding that the relationship still exists at law.

After the decision, Gerald continued to pay child support. The Pennsylvania Supreme Court affirmed the lower court ruling in 1998.

In many ways, *Miscovich v. Miscovich* is a thoroughly modern case. Gerald seized on DNA testing as a revolutionary technology that promised to provide a scientific precision in disputed paternity cases that was previously unimaginable, and one that might finally protect men from an ancient form of victimization. It would, though, do much more. Resort to DNA testing in child custody disputes by men like Gerald raises fundamental questions about how the law defines parental responsibility and children's interests. It does so in heartbreaking stories of clashing claims of victimization involving adulterous wives, duped dads, and discarded children.

Family law scholar Carol Sanger has identified the significance of these newly emergent conflicts. "Now that DNA testing has washed off the table the reasons we didn't use to allow paternity evidence, we have to decide whether there are other reasons to keep that evidence out, like child support and fairness," Sanger explained to a newspaper reporter. There are, she contended, "real concerns about letting biology trump all. The state may want to make sure that if they take one dad off the hook, they will have another one paying. The underlying question is, what establishes a parental relationship?" (quoted in Lewin 2001). Complicating the issues, she maintained, is the reality that any policy that emphasizes biological ties could upset the nascent recognition of nontraditional families, such as same-sex partnerships, and that children may suffer from the disruption of their ties to a father figure. Yet, as in all family law problems, those concerns must be balanced with others. Sanger admitted that, for some experts, any legal policy that did not acknowledge scientific truth would be disturbing, especially at a time when criminal courts are allowing people to use DNA evidence to prove their innocence no matter how long after a crime. "Its real question: if we let DNA do its work in the criminal justice system, why not in the family court system?" said Sanger. Yet, she insists, the "answer is that the concerns are different. We never want an innocent person in jail. But to put it in the most melodramatic way, in the paternity situation, children are the innocent party. While some people might see the refusal to accept DNA evidence of nonpaternity as rewarding the wife for deception, I think courts look at its use as punishing the children" (Lewin 2001). As Sanger's comments make clear, both the modernity and the future implications of DNA testing are obvious and obviously important.

Despite its modernity, *Miscovich v. Miscovich* has an equally consequential past. It is a history that highlights changing conceptions of the American family and changing notions of the social and legal significance of biological ties in parent-child relationships. DNA testing brings this past into the present, because it forces to the surface some persistent tensions in American family life and law. Identifying and understanding those tensions can help us understand the problems this new technology poses for children, women, and men today. Making this past useable in the present requires going back to the mid eighteenth century and interrogating the reigning paradigm in North American and European family history—the modern family. This new type of household not only spawned new family forms, practices, and beliefs, it also sparked debates about how families should be organized and governed.

All of these are still with us in the twenty-first century, and two are critical for understanding the issues raised by DNA testing in child custody cases: evolving definitions of a fit parent and changing conceptions of paternal responsibility. They have interlocking but separate histories that are best recounted by dividing their pasts into two distinct eras: a long-ago nineteenth century and a more recent twentieth century. Giving DNA testing a past by placing disputes such as *Miscovich v. Miscovich* in historical context will not solve the problems raised by this new technology. But it will help us understand more fully the nature and implications of the policy choices that must be made when we devise guidelines for using DNA testing in child custody.

Nineteenth-Century Transformations

The modern family emerged as a result of radical changes in North American and European households in the late eighteenth and early nineteenth centuries. At the heart of those changes was a fundamental transformation of the family that jettisoned lingering colonial practices that treated the home as a corporate entity presided over by a powerful patriarch and linked it directly to the larger community. In its place emerged a conception of the family as a refuge from society and as a collection of distinct individuals bound together by choice and emotional bonds. The radical implications of these changes meant that lingering traditional household commitments such as property rights and blood ties were placed in a significantly altered context. Critically, as family historians have described in detail, the new family beliefs and practices treated children, more than ever before, as distinct individuals with special needs and interests and treated childhood as a distinct phase of life. These beliefs in turn helped to elevate the importance of the mother-child bond, made child nurture more directly a fundamental maternal responsibility, and enhanced the importance of the home as a nursery for future citizens and workers. Central to these developments were changes in the definition of a fit parent and paternal responsibility and clashes over their meaning (Mintz and Kellogg 1988).

Fit Parents

The changes sparked by the advent of the modern family were so monumental that a new legal definition of a fit parent had to be devised. It emerged most directly out of clashes over child custody. Traditionally, Anglo-American law deemed custody a patriarchal prerogative. In the corporate household, the patriarch exchanged maintenance and education of his offspring for the right to their custody and service. Those rights were seldom challenged. However, the new family upset these arrangements and provoked challenges to paternal custody rights, particularly by mothers. The contests took place primarily when marriages fell apart and spouses used newly legitimate and accessible laws of separation and divorce to settle child placement. Like DNA testing in the early twenty-first century, these spousal disputes in the nineteenth century forced to the surface conflicting notions of fit parents. The most significant result was the emergence of "social parenting"—a definition of a fit parent that identified child nurture as the most significant parental skill and responsibility. The creation of social parenting was critical because it has, ever since, helped frame legal and social debates about who gets the child in a custody dispute. In particular, the reliance on social parenting has led to a constantly expanding notion of a fit parent, which has meant that the quality of child care has become an increasingly important, fundamental factor in legal determinations of child placement. Social parenting thus became a key component of the legal rules and practices that would emerge in disputes about the use of DNA testing in child custody cases.

Social parenting emerged early in the nineteenth century as family change forced policy makers to reformulate their approach to custody disputes. Their search for new ways to balance parental rights and filial needs found its most revealing result in a legal phrase that would dominate legal debates about children into the twenty-first century: *the best interests of the child.* Though the exact origins of the phrase are not clear, judges and other policy makers translated the traditional power of *parens patriae* of the state as the guardian of all dependents and the newfound sense of children as having distinct interests into the *best interests* expression. As a Georgia superior court judge declared in an 1836 child custody case, "All legal rights, even those of personal security and liberty, may be forfeited by improper conduct, and so this legal right of the father to the possession of his child must be made subservient to the true interests and safety of the child, and the duty of the State to protect its citizens of whatever age" (*In the Matter of Mitchell* 1836). The ambiguous phrase assumed separate children's needs yet expressed the conviction that others— most appropriately parents and, when they failed, judges or other suitable public or private officials such as the overseers of the poor—must determine them. It sanctioned broad discretionary authority to determine the interests of children when family conflicts or failures made them disorderly or dependent. In particular, it gave judges wide discretionary power to define child welfare and evaluate parental fitness, which in turn made custody case narratives battles over stories of good and bad fathers, mothers, and guardians. In this way, the new doctrine retained the traditional belief in the sanctity of blood ties and the assumption that biological ties provided the most secure, indeed the most natural, source of parental concern for the young. But it also opened the legal door for expanding notions of social parenting by stressing the nurturing needs of children, thereby launching debates on the meaning and scope of social parenting that continue to this day.

The most far-reaching result of this new set of concerns and balances in the law was the institutionalization of maternal preference as the dominant rule in custody law. Over the course of the nineteenth century, judges constructed the new rule as changes in gender roles led mothers in collapsing marriages to claim their children. Mothers and their lawyers argued successfully that child care was fundamentally an issue of nurture and that women were naturally endowed with the requisite skills. Treatise writer James Schouler explained the new consensus in an early-twentieth-century revision of his widely used compilation of American domestic relations law: "The physical, moral, and spiritual welfare of the child is the only safe guide in cases of the custody of a child in divorce proceedings. The love of the mother for her child, regardless of condition and environment, has been proven by the history of the ages, and while her devotion can be counted upon unfailingly, it is sad to say that sometimes the tie between father and child is a different matter, and requires the strong arm of the law to regulate it with some degree of humanity and tenderness for the child's good" (Schouler 1906, 2:2034–35). Those convictions ensured that the definition of a fit parent led to maternal custody (Grossberg 1985).

Equally significant, judges constructed collateral custody rules that also gave primacy to child nurture. Particularly important for questions of parental fitness and paternal responsibility was the established ties rule. Through this rule, American courts in the nineteenth century gave increasing weight to the interests of children in staying with those who reared them. Thus in 1881 the Kansas Supreme Court turned aside a claim from a man attempting to recover custody of his biological daughter from the sister of his late wife, who had raised the child for more than five years: "When new ties have been formed and a certain current given to the child's life and thought, much attention should be paid to the probabilities of a benefit to the child from the change. It is an obvious fact, that ties of blood weaken, and ties of companionship strengthen, by lapse of time; and the prosperity and welfare of the child depend on the ability to do all which the prompting of these ties compels" (*Chapsky v. Wood* 1881).

The radical potential of the new nurture-based ideal of parental fitness to reorder custody law also emerged in the transformation of illegitimacy and the creation of adoption. Bastards, as Anglo-American law had long classified children born out of wedlock, faced legal repression and discrimination. Statutes, doctrines, and customs used matrimony to separate legal from spurious issue. The latter suffered the legal status of *filius nullius,* the child and heir of no one, which meant that the bastard had no recognized legal relations with his or her parents and no claims to inheritance, maintenance, or family membership. Nor did the illicit couple have any rights or duties toward the child. The English reluctance to help bastards was evident in the refusal to follow the civil law and allow legitimation by the subsequent marriage of the parents. The only major reform in the law came with the inclusion of bastards in the Elizabethan Poor Law and the demand that parents aid in their upkeep, but this reform sought to protect taxpayers' pocketbooks not to provide child nurture. The traditional bastardy law had two primary purposes: repelling challenges to established family organization, especially property distribution, and preventing the public from being saddled with the costs of rearing children born out of wedlock. Beyond streamlining paternity hearings, colonial Americans seem to have made few alterations in the law (Grossberg 1985; O'Donovan 1988).

After the Revolution, however, many Americans began to question the logic of bastardy law. Thomas Jefferson, for example, argued that children should not be punished for the sins of their parents. This new idea of child innocence has had a continuing resonance with succeeding generations of Americans and is one of the fundamental concerns that that has emerged in debates on DNA testing. In the 1790s it led Jefferson to promote revisions in Virginia law that reduced the chance of being designated a bastard. Statutes and judicial decisions in Virginia and then throughout the republic declared the offspring of a couple who wed after its birth to be legitimate. They did the same for the children of annulled marriages (Grossberg 1999). The new logic was evident in the case *Stones v. Keeling* (1804). William Keeling had married Arthalia Arbuckle while her first husband was still living. They had a daughter; William had a son from his first marriage. When Keeling died, the son and daughter fought over his estate, with the son challenging the girl's legitimacy. In 1804, Virginia judges cast aside that challenge: "a strong case to show the sense of the legislature that the turpitude or guilt of the marriage should not break upon the heads of their innocent offspring."

That same notion of protecting innocent children by expanding the definition of a fit parent led judges to create a new legal household and bind it together with inheritance rights by turning the customary bonds between the bastard and his or her mother into a web of reciprocal legal rights and duties. The judiciary granted such women custody rights in a reinterpretation of the law that combined the new faith in maternal care with a postrevolutionary assertion of judicial authority over the allocation of domestic rights and responsibilities. Similarly, judges and legislators began to confer reciprocal inheritance rights on bastards and their mothers and on other kin. As a result of this dramatic expansion of the legal definition of a fit parent, the bastard began to have his or her own set of rights and responsibilities, as legislators and judges relied on new notions of the welfare of the child and the rights of the mother to sever family membership from the punishment for sexual immorality and property protection (Grossberg 1985).

The creation of legal adoption was an even more dramatic example of the radical potential of the new ideas of a fit parent. It dissolved the "natural" (blood) ties of family relation and replaced them with the "artificial" (legal) ties of kinship. English law, with its priorities of family preservation and property protection, had never recognized the possibility of such a change; indeed, the English would not accept adoption until 1926. Only apprenticeship, which gave a master parental-like powers and responsibilities, allowed for the legal transfer of child custody under English law. However, the new nineteenth-century custody law regime in the United States encouraged this radical innovation of parent-child relations based on choice, not birth, and on nurture, not blood. Massachusetts enacted the first modern adoption law in 1851. It created a judicially supervised parental transfer of custodial rights from natural to adopted parents. Relying on now widely accepted notions of social parenting, judges were charged with ensuring that adoptive parents had "sufficient ability to bring up the child" and that the adoption was "fit and proper." "The heart of the adoption transfer," Jamil Zainaldin explains in identifying the centrality of social parenting in the new legal relationship, "became the judicially monitored transfer of rights with due regard for the welfare of the child and the parental qualifications of the adopters" (Zainaldin 1979, 1043).

By the end of the nineteenth century, adoption had been enacted in every state. This rapid diffusion revealed the widespread conviction that the republic had the responsibility to provide a nurturing and stable environment for children who lost their homes as a result of parental death, poverty, or neglect. It also expressed the determination to offer poor law officials permanent relief from their obligations to supervise the welfare of such children. These beliefs gradually overcame the initial resistance to severing the traditional English common law connection between bloodlines and inheritance rights and made adoption a central feature of American social welfare and family law. As the Tennessee Supreme Court observed, "It is difficult to see, upon any rule of construction, or of policy, why all the powers possessed by a natural father should not be exercised by him, who, by adoption of a minor, assumes the relationship of a parent" (quoted in Grossberg 1985, 275; Carp 1998).

The rise of maternal preference, the transformation of bastardy law, and the creation of adoption suggest the expansive nature of the legal definition of a fit parent occurring in this era. The changes were rooted in the new belief that custody law must recognize the importance of children's innocence and distinctive needs. The new rules also demonstrated the radical power of such beliefs to rearrange family legal rights and duties.

The transformation of custody law, however, did not completely eliminate traditional concerns. As always, continuity existed along with change and revealed some of its limits. For example, though appealing in many ways, adoption remained a secondary type of family formation. Acting as a counterweight to the broad acceptance of adoption was the continuing belief in blood as the only completely legitimate basis for kinship. The inferior status of adoption was evident in popular discourse. Adoptive parents were contrasted with "natural" or "normal" ones. Discriminatory laws reinforced the notion that the adoptive relationship was inherently flawed. For instance, jurists regularly ruled in inheritance cases that adoption violated the legal principle of consanguinity. In practice, this meant that adopted children did not have the same inheritance rights as birth children. Indeed, inheritance not custody was the most litigated issue involving adoption. And in other cases dealing with disputed custody rights of adopted children, both courts and legislatures favored natural parents' appeals to restore their children to them. Such policies suggested the treatment of adoption as a social welfare measure as much as a family formation device.

The uncertain status of adoption was also apparent in attempts to make the new households resemble those created through blood. In the 1920s, state officials began "sealing" adoption records. The original birth certificate was placed out of public reach, and an amended birth certificate naming the adoptive parents as the birth parents replaced it. Social workers and others who oversaw the creation of adoptive families developed the practice of "matching":

selecting adoptees based on their racial, religious, and physical resemblance to prospective adopters. The goal was to make the adoptive family "look" real (O'Donovan 1988). Efforts to approximate blood families narrowed the definition of a fit parent by giving priority to resemblance over social parenting. They also underscore the continued importance of biological ties in legal definitions of parent-child relations (Grossberg 1985; Carp 1998).

Even though such limits existed, by the early twentieth century a nurture-dominated child custody law regime had become American legal orthodoxy. With it came a radical redefinition of a fit parent, one that gave legal preference to mothers and created an expanding ideal of social parenting. Developed during the nineteenth century, these innovations framed discussions about child custody well into the twentieth century.

Paternal Responsibility

As the transformation of the legal definition of fit parenthood suggests, the diminution of the parental role of fathers was central to the new family. In colonial America, as in early modern Europe, the father had been the primary parent and played a critical role in all aspects of his children's lives. The modern family, by contrast, with its sharply distinguished gender roles and separation from the larger society, undermined paternal authority, first in middle-class homes and then among other classes. Linked to the emergence of market capitalism, the modern family experienced a sharp disconnection of work from the home, as farming became more technological and market driven and declined as a percentage of the economy in favor of shops, factories, and professions. These economic changes took men from their homes and undermined their parental responsibilities, while reinforcing the primary role of mothers as children's caregivers. Though men retained their position as heads of household and served as primary family disciplinarians, the combination of economic change and the rise of the nurturing ideal of fit parenthood made the role of fathers in child care problematic. Indeed, historian Robert Griswold concludes that "as the [nineteenth] century came to a close, fathers were becoming increasingly marginal within the home itself" (Griswold 1993, 33).

The redefinition of fatherhood in the construction of the modern family made breadwinning—a term coined in early-nineteenth-century America—the fundamental paternal responsibility (Kimmel 1997). Of course, male fiscal responsibility was hardly new. Nor was male evasion of family support a modern phenomenon; it, too, has a long history in North America and Europe, as did lax enforcement (Willrich 2000). But as breadwinning became the singular definition of a responsible father, the determination arose to make men accountable for paternal responsibilities. It made breadwinning the primary subject of legal debate and dispute involving fathers. Not surprisingly, this issue, too, would reemerge in debates about DNA testing.

Custody law is a prime example of the fundamental redefinition of paternal responsibilities that led to declining male parental authority and rising economic responsibilities. Holding that children were the responsibility of fathers, Anglo-American courts had traditionally given fathers custody of children when marital disputes split families. The new attitudes toward motherhood and children led jurists to argue that fathers' right to custody was only presumptive and could be overcome if children's interests were better served by staying with their mothers. And the institutionalization of maternal preference in custody law compelled courts to abandon the very idea of a father's presumptive right. Instead, judges maintained that custody decisions should be based on the best interests of the child, the standard that emphasized social parenting and thus maternal care. Following such reasoning and invoking what would be called the tender years rule, the California Supreme Court decided in 1860 that mothers should raise young children and girls when spousal conflict forced parents apart: "That a child of the tender age of this could be better cared for by the mother, with whom she could be almost constantly, than the father, whose necessary avocations would withdraw him, in great measure, from personal superintendence, is plain enough" (*Wand v. Wand* 1860). Other courts argued that the presumptive right of custody ultimately resided with mothers.

The expansion of state services also eroded the formerly preeminent position of fathers. Beginning in the 1830s and 1840s, a variety of public institutions emerged to perform health, education, and welfare duties formerly carried out in the home and overseen by fathers. The common school movement increasingly made education a public responsibility. New institutions to care for vagrant, incorrigible, neglected, and impoverished children also replaced family care. According to the Pennsylvania Supreme Court, in a seminal decision that turned back a father's challenge to the incarceration of his daughter in the state house of refuge, "To this end, may not the natural parents, when unequal to the task of education or unworthy of it, be superseded by the *parens patriae*, or common guardianship of the community?" (*Ex parte Crouse* 1839). With these rulings, the right to custody, once an almost absolute paternal prerogative, could now be lost much more easily if a father misused his authority. And paternal power receded further with the imposition of compulsory school laws and child labor regulations that restricted fathers' power to decide when a child should enter the workforce and contribute to the family economy. Juvenile courts added yet another level of legal surveillance that undermined the parental autonomy of fathers.

Changes in custody law and public authority rendered fathers secondary if not suspect parents, who were presumed incompetent as child rearers and responsible only for family support. These developments created a new sense of male victimization that also became part of the dynamics of the modern family—as did male resistance to taking responsibility for the care and support of children. The reduced parental role, sense of victimization, and tradition of evasion, all of which are central to the contemporary response of men to DNA testing, emerged over the course of the nineteenth century as breadwinning became the focus of legal disputes about paternity, support after divorce, and desertion. Critically, concern about breadwinning highlighted blood ties as the most legitimate basis for paternal responsibility and thus clashed with the trend to define parental fitness in terms of nurture and social parenting. It also strengthened the conviction that without evidence of biological links between father and child, men had no responsibility for children.

These realities were apparent in clashes over the traditional vehicle for determining child support: paternity hearings. The inquiries were grounded in fundamental gender realities: unlike the biological relation between mother and child, the biological relation between father and child was impossible to ascertain with any certainty. At the heart of paternity hearings, then, was the ancient problem of how to find fathers when men refused to come forward. The preoccupation of the hearings with paternal support underscored the state's vital interest in fixing paternity on some man and thus obtaining child support. Statutes relied on paternal support obligations to protect the state and its unwed mothers from the economic burdens of rearing bastards. In doing so, the law held the community and the mother as victims of male lust and irresponsibility. And given the parsimonious child welfare programs, finding a fiscally responsible adult was critical for a child's well-being if not survival (Grossberg 1985).

Paternity hearings, like their subject, were bastardized legal creations. Postrevolutionary judges repeatedly insisted on classifying them as civil proceedings, but they retained the trappings of criminal trials because of their dual objectives of determining paternity and compelling support. A Kentucky man discovered the implications of this mixture in 1809, when the state Supreme Court rejected his plea that men arraigned on bastardy charges be granted the rights of defendants in a criminal trial: "the case of bastardy cannot be considered as a criminal prosecution; nor the order for the maintenance of the child, in the nature of a criminal penalty." Instead, the judges asserted the nineteenth-century version of traditional paternalism: the "true object of the law seems to be, to enforce upon the unfeeling father, the performance of a natural duty for the easement and benefit of the mother, at whose instance the prosecution be instituted or carried on" (*Schnooner v. Commonwealth* 1809).

The hybrid nature of bastardy proceedings eased the most vexing problem facing local authorities: identifying the father. The need to do so to secure child maintenance was balanced by the recognition that men could easily be victimized by false accusations and tenuous evidence. Colonials had treated a woman's accusation as tantamount to conviction, particularly in the folk belief that a woman asked about the father of her child at the moment of birth could not lie. Similarly, most American courts relied on "bald eagle tests": the belief that resemblance proved paternity (*State v. Bowles* 1860; *Gilmantown v. Ham* 1859; *Wright v. Hicks* 1854; *Clark v. Bradstreet* 1888; Doering 1925–26; Shapiro, Reifler, and Psome 1992–93). But these customary legal tools were less and less appealing in the rights-conscious new republic. The hearings usually boiled down to accusatory battles between former lovers. Because these were considered civil proceedings, the woman merely had to establish a preponderance of the evidence in favor of paternity. The right of the parties to testify did, however, represent a gradual change in the rights of the litigants. In this type of suit, as in many others, the old common law prohibition of the testimony of interested parties faded away. The new conviction that justice demanded the presentation of all relevant information fueled the change. Thus in 1849 the Supreme Court of North Carolina instructed one putative father, "You may, if you please, submit the question of your guilt to a jury, but if you do so, the burden of showing your innocence shall be on you; for the examination of the woman shall be sufficient to convict you, unless you show that you are not the father of the child" (*State v. Goode* 1849). By transforming paternity into an issue of fact to be determined by a jury, authorities had gone as far as they would in balancing paternal rights with community interests.

Dwindling faith in traditional methods of identifying biological fathers, combined with men's claims of victimization and the powerful nineteenth-century belief in fault as the only legitimate basis for individual legal responsibility, led to persistent attempts to find a reliable paternity test. Its most significant success came with the development of paternity blood tests by Dr. Karl Landsteiner at the University of Vienna in 1901. The early blood tests could only exclude potential fathers, they could not identify the biological father of a particular child. By the 1930s, judges and legislators began to accept test results as evidence. The development of blood tests encouraged the continued search for a scientifically valid paternity identification technology, while reinforcing the belief that men should be responsible only for children proven to be their biological offspring (Glennon 2000).

Throughout the nineteenth century and into the twentieth, however, neither traditional techniques nor new technology could identify the biological father of a child with anything approaching complete certainty. This biological reality encouraged a continued reliance on the presumption of paternity that would reappear years later in cases such as *Miscovich v. Miscovich*. After the Revolution, all states adopted the traditional policy that husbands were presumed to be the fathers of children conceived or born during their marriage. Only evidence that the husband was sterile, impotent, or lacked access to his wife could be used to challenge the presumption. American judges and legislators also adopted Lord Mansfield's exclusionary rule of 1777, which decreed "the declarations of a father or mother, [can] not be admitted to bastardize the issue born after the marriage." Mere evidence of a husband's absence, therefore, could not be used to bastardize a child born to his wife; only uncontroverted evidence could do so (*Michigan Law Review* 1930).

Particularly in an age before blood tests, the difficulty of proving paternity and the presumption of legitimacy granted to children born in wedlock meant that the judicial refusal to allow a married couple to testify on the question reinforced both ends of bastardy law. It protected children from illegitimacy and helped local officials guard their purses. Accordingly, family law scholar Janet Dolgin maintains, "Before the advent of paternity testing, courts were able to apply the presumption without confronting biological evidence proving that the presumption failed utterly to reflect the biological facts of paternity. As a result, the presumption rarely collided irrefutably with alternative facts" (Dolgin 2000, 528). The rule, though, could well collide with the knowledge of the spouses. Historian Norma Basch argues in her study of divorce in nineteenth-century America that "men's suits . . . frequently pivoted on the thorny problem of paternity. Indeed, in these divorce records male anxiety about paternity is pervasive" (Basch 1999, 136). Thus in the agonizing conflict between a man's right to limit his paternity only to his actual offspring and the right of a child born to a married woman to claim family membership, the common law, first in England and then in America, generally made paternal rights defer to the larger goal of preserving family integrity.

Judges also invoked the innocence of children to justify the rule. New York Chancellor Rueben Walworth did so in 1831: "It becomes the duty of the court to examine those proofs with the most rigid scrutiny in order to prevent the rights of innocent children from being sacrificed by the misconduct or negligence of their parents." Accepting that the four seas rule should no longer prevail, he nonetheless argued that "the modern rule, which has been marked out by its good sense, is that to bastardize the issue of a married woman, it must be shown beyond all reasonable doubt that there was no such access as could have enabled the husband to be the father of the child" (*Cross v. Cross* 1831). Adulterine bastardy stood condemned as one of the most reprehensible acts a wife could commit, but her punishment remained separate from that of her child.

Over the course of the nineteenth century, judges in both the United States and Britain gradually widened the acceptable range of evidence that could be offered by spouses and placed restraints on the nonaccess rule. Nevertheless, the presumption was always a disputed doctrine and fed a sense of male victimization. The rule also ignored the growing conviction of jurists and legal scholars that litigants had the right to present all evidence supporting their causes. Indeed, John Wigmore, the late nineteenth century's reigning authority on the law of evidence, insisted that Lord Mansfield had created a doctrine without the aid of precedent, the perennial complaint of lawyers when policy is at issue. Wigmore argued that in bastardy cases, as in other litigation, all the pertinent facts should be admitted. He condemned as absurd and unwise the inability of married persons to compile and present the full evidence on the question of access. Wigmore contended that the rule allowed immorality and indecency under the pretext of preventing them: "The truth is that these high sounding 'decencies' and 'moralities' are mere phrasical afterthoughts, invented to explain an otherwise incomprehensible rule and there is just as little reason or policy to maintain it" (Wigmore 1904, 2:2768). But Wigmore found few allies, because such disputes pitted the rights and interests of family members and the state against each other. In turn-of-the-century America the doctrine still served the law's larger purposes of limiting bastardy and protecting children.

The dogged determination to establish paternity was matched by a determination to ensure that men fulfilled their breadwinning duties as fathers. Campaigns arose to compel men to fulfill financial obligations ordered in divorce decrees and to catch men who deserted their wives and children. Both would be recurrent features of modern American family policy. Critically, both were rooted in another emerging characteristic of the modern family and its law: the separation of support from custody. Over the course of the nineteenth century, legislators and judges decided that maintenance and custody were no longer mutually dependent rights. Instead, in yet another expression of the pervasive impact of the breadwinning role on men's lives, they decreed that a father must support his children even if he lost custody (Mason 1994). The consequences were evident in policies toward illegitimate children. Unlike in colonial America, where a father could elect to raise a child rather than give support to his or her mother, under the new best-interests-of-the-child regime fathers had to support their illegitimate children but had no claim to custody (*Hudson v. Hills* 1836). Separating support and custody fed a sense of unfairness that led many men to resist support orders.

At the same time, the massive increase in divorce during the nineteenth century created a critical new legal terrain for paternal responsibility. As the legal dissolution of marriage became more common, judges and legislators devised policies in a family law regime whose rigid gender ideology encouraged women to stay out of the workplace and defined men as breadwinners. Thus, as in the decision to separate child support from custody, judges began to separate matrimony from spousal support, as the logic of the breadwinning conception of paternal responsibility led them to make men more financially accountable to their cast-off wives as well as to their discarded children. Accordingly, the Texas Supreme Court declared in 1926, "the primary duty to support rests on the father since human experience demonstrates that he is best able to perform the duty" (*Milburn v. Milburn* 1923).

Lawmakers were even less solicitous of men who deserted their families. In the new regime of the modern family, male desertion became one of the most grievous offenses a husband or father could commit. Early in the twentieth century, social workers, philanthropists, judges, and other reformers attacked these men with newly coined epithets: "delinquent husbands"; "married vagabonds"; "worthless men"; and "home slackers." Public concern about what seemed like a tidal wave of male desertion, concerns fed by fears of irresponsible immigrant men, led every state to rewrite its laws between 1890 and 1915. They imposed higher fines or longer jail terms for husbands who failed to support their wives and children. Many made nonsupport a felony rather than a misdemeanor. States also allowed deserted wives to testify against their husbands in court, something previously impossible because coverture rendered such testimony as self-incrimination, the two spouses being legally one person. Lillian Brandt, a New York charity worker, said in 1905, "The chief value of a good law, well enforced is that it expresses the estimation in which society holds men who shirk their obligations to their families, and that it relieves society of the necessity of assuming their responsibilities" (quoted in May 1988, 47). Criminalization, regulation, and punishment of able-bodied male breadwinners who failed to support their families meant that male prerogatives authorized by the breadwinner norm were made conditional on men fulfilling their assigned roles. As the Kansas Supreme Court made clear in upholding one of the new laws, "The essence of the act is that a man shall not be allowed to shift the burden of supporting his wife and children upon others under no obligation to bear it, and possibly upon the state itself" (*State v. Waller* 1913).

New legal policies and definitions of fit parents and paternal responsibility were developed during the nineteenth century as legal components of the modern family. Though modified, they continued to govern American homes well into the twentieth century. Significantly, the expansion of fit parenthood and the contraction of paternal responsibility were complementary developments, but also ones that could conflict with each other. They thus produced tensions and uncertainties that bubbled beneath the surface of American family life and law.

Late–Twentieth-Century Revisions

A second era of family law transformation occurred in the second half of the twentieth century. Though not completely revamped, the family law regime that had been constructed during the nineteenth century and the first part of the twentieth century was revised in significant ways. Examples of the fundamental changes in the law range from the advent of no-fault divorce and surrogate motherhood to the legalization of abortion and interracial marriage. Amid these changes, conceptions of fit parenthood and paternal responsibility were transformed as well. At the same time, the development of DNA testing in child custody cases brought to the surface lingering conflicts about the constitution of American families and the rights, responsibilities, and interests of its members, which has led to a search for a new orthodoxy in custody law (Grossberg 2000).

Parental Fitness

The legal definition of a fit parent expanded further in the second half of the twentieth century as the law of child custody underwent a transformation almost as great as in the early nineteenth century. Expansion came as a result of the repudiation of key assumptions and policies crafted in the previous era. In another period of major changes in gender roles and beliefs, the central tenet of custody rules—maternalism—came under attack as an ideal and a policy. Support for the presumed superior ability of mothers to raise children that undergirded the law began to erode. Psychologist Arlene Skolnick summarized the situation by explaining that maternal preference had "remained unchallenged until the family upheavals of the 1960s and 1970s. In the wake of rising divorce rates, challenges to women's traditional roles, and men's claims of sex discrimination in custody awards, most states abandoned the maternal presumption in favor of a more gender neutral 'best-interests' standard" (Skolnick 1998, 242). Such sentiments shifted the balance of power between mothers and fathers. Though most awards of physical custody went to women, the new rules enabled more fathers to secure custody than ever before. They also led to new custodial arrangements such as joint custody, shared custody, and divided custody. All of these would have been unthinkable in the previous family law regime (Mason 1994).

Most important for understanding the debate about DNA testing, the rejection of maternal preference forced a search for new legal definitions of fit parents. Custody law became one of the most divisive and visible legal battlegrounds in an era when family law often dominated the public sphere and always dominated civil court dockets. The popularity of the Oscar-winning film *Kramer versus Kramer,* which pitted a nurturing father in a custody battle against his wife, who had abandoned her family but then returned to reclaim her maternal rights and duties, revealed the compelling nature of child custody conflicts and the new and uncertain legal and social terrain on which they were waged. As the film dramatized, the elimination of maternal preference reopened the question of what constituted a fit parent and of the place and meaning of social parenting in custody law. There have been no stable and permanent answers; indeed, the debate has carried into the early twenty-first century, making it one of the complications in devising widely acceptable rules about DNA testing in custody cases.

Nevertheless, some of the consequences of regime change have become apparent. Fathers, for instance, have benefited from the demise of maternal preference. Their legal power and roles in families expanded for the first time in the history of the modern family. Indeed, antimaternalism arose in part from the first major questioning of the assumption that women were natural child rearers and, its converse, that men were not. Beginning most obviously in the "antimomism" complaints of the 1950s, some social critics began to argue that a female-dominated parental regime was bad for boys in particular and deprived both girls and boys of needed fatherly guidance and male role models (Kimmel 1997). Arguments about the importance of dads reinforced complementary gender changes that encouraged male and female equality in custody law.

The most dramatic and far-reaching impact of the revived legal recognition of fathers was evident in changes in notions of paternal responsibility, as discussed below, but changes in custody law also widened the legal definition of a fit parent by encouraging challenges to all parental rights claims, not only gendered ones. In the process, social parenting—the importance of child nurture as the fundamental role of a parent—received new support. One of the most influential developments was the use of social science theories such as the "psychological parent" to buttress the custody claims of caregivers. That theory propounded that children always became attached to one individual, though not necessarily the biological parent. Indeed, such theories supported the continued role of women as the default parent despite the legal revisions. Belief in such theories, for instance, led a Denver judge to tell *Time* magazine, "In my courtroom, they stay where they've been nurtured. You have to consider who the child feels is the psychological parent. If you have a good bond in that home, I'm not about to break it" (quoted in Skolnick 1998, 253). These sentiments also encouraged the expansion of social parenting by highlighting the importance of effective child care. Perhaps the most dramatic evidence of this expanding notion of parental fitness came from the increasing acceptance of gay and lesbian couples as parents. In Massachusetts, for instance, the Supreme Judicial Court ruled that homosexual partners could be capable, loving parents and therefore interpreted the adoption statute to allow joint adoption by same-sex couples (*Adoption of Tammy* 1993). And in another case the same court concluded that a prospective adopting couple being of the same sex was irrelevant to their fitness as prospective parents (*Adoption of Galen* 1997).

Debates on the expansion of social parenting occurred primarily in custody disputes involving adoption, foster care, and stepparents. Significantly, each of these was a parent-child relationship based on choice not blood and thus directly raised questions about the legal standing of social parenting.

Expansion was certainly the theme of adoption in the second half of the twentieth century. The numbers of adoptive families grew significantly after World War II as postwar prosperity, a pronatalist climate of opinion, and medical advances in infertility diagnosis combined to produce a remarkable increase in the number of applications to adopt a child. From 1945 to 1965 the number of adoptions grew nearly ninefold, to 142,000. Adoption also gained new social acceptance and that, in turn, helped expand the range of adoptable children and thus fit parents. The population of adoptable children became more inclusive as social workers, parents, and others involved in adoption became less fixated on the need to match the physical, mental, racial, and religious characteristics of adopted children and adoptive parents. The decline of matching led to an expanding definition of adoptable children that for the first time came to include disabled, minority, older, and foreign-born children. Though many of these children remained without adoptive families, expansion signaled a movement away from the determination to make adopted families replicate biological ones. At the same time, federal policy, most notably the Adoption and Safe Families Act of 1997 (Public Law 105-89, 111 *Stat.* 2115), expressed a preference for adoption when children were found to be in abusive homes or were left by parents in foster families.

Nevertheless, in many ways adoption remained "a form of second-rate kinship." This was evident in the 1970s with the emergence of the adoption rights movement. Adoption rights activists, composed mostly of adult adopted persons and birth mothers, demanded the right to identifying information in the adoption record. They campaigned to repeal sealed records laws. Equally significant was the effort of groups such as the National Association of Black Social Workers to ban adoption across racial lines in the United States, on the grounds that it constituted a form of racial genocide for African Americans and that white families could not provide an effective "safety net" against the racism their black children would certainly experience (Carp 1998; Bartholet

1999). As sociologists Dorothy Nelkin and Susan Lindee observed, "The pre-occupation with genetic relationships can stigmatize the experience of adoption; make it seem like a last resort, debased form of parenting, coin phrases like real or natural parents versus unnatural substitutes; opponents call adoption a pathology and argue that genetics is the basis of identity, and say that adoptees are amputees" (Nelkin and Lindee 1995, 70–71). The persistent debate about the legitimacy of adoption reinforced the significance of blood ties in legal definitions of fit parents, despite the growing significance of social parenting.

The dominance of foster care as the state's preferred placement for orphaned, neglected, and abused children also reinforced social parenting as a central definition of a fit parent. In theory, foster homes served as a temporary respite before return to family or adoption, but in reality many children spent much of their childhood in foster care. State-licensed and subject to regulations on the size of home, number of children, and age of parents, foster families received fees in exchange for child care. Their contracts stipulated that the legal responsibility for the child remained with the agency, which had the right to terminate the foster relationship. In effect, foster mothers and fathers became licensed social parents—a significantly less legally endowed role than the one assumed by masters in the traditional apprentice system of child placement (Mason 1994).

Despite their importance in the modern American welfare state, foster parents lacked the rights of parents. Children could be removed from their homes even though strong emotional bonds had been formed. Like others in a rights-conscious age, foster parents turned to the courts for relief. The most important response came from the U.S. Supreme Court in the 1977 decision of *Smith v. Organization of Foster Families for Equality and Reform*. The justices heard the pleas of foster parents who claimed that they had a constitutionally protected liberty interest in the children they cared for and thus the right to demand a full hearing before those children were removed from their care. In effect, foster parents grasped the now entrenched custody doctrine of established ties to try to garb themselves with greater parental rights. The justices offered them some solace by emphasizing the importance of social parenting: "The importance of the familial relationship, to the individuals involved and to the society, stems from the emotional attachments that derive from the intimacy of daily association, and from the role it plays in 'promoting a way of life' through the instruction of children, as well as from the fact of blood relationship . . . for this reason we cannot dismiss the foster family as a mere collection of unrelated individuals." Nevertheless, the Court sanctioned the secondary legal status of foster families. Justice William J. Brennan expressed a continued commitment to protect the rights of natural parents who had not fully relinquished their children: "The usual understanding of 'family' implies biological relationships, and most decisions treating the relationship between parent and child have stressed that element" (*Smith v. Organization* 1977).

Stepparents, inheritors of an equally problematic legal status, also grew in numbers as divorce, remarriage, and even redivorce became more common. Yet, like foster parents, they too had significant child care responsibilities without commensurate parental rights. As legal scholar Wendy Mahoney contended in a study of stepparents, "A major purpose of many family-related doctrines is to safeguard the interests of individual family members, especially children, and also to protect the family unit. The traditional emphasis on the nuclear family has effectively prevented many individuals, who live in other family situations, from enjoying the same type of legal recognition and protection" (Mahoney 1994, 1). Indeed, after documenting the hold of the past on the present, Mahoney bleakly concluded that the transformations of the era had left the rights of stepparents virtually unchanged, even though the surging divorce rate produced more and more of them. Mason explained the consequences of this legal reality: "The revolution in divorce and custody laws that swept through the states in the late twentieth century almost totally ignored the growing presence of stepparents. Family law continued to view stepparents through common law lenses, giving them no legal rights over their stepchildren and imposing few obligations" (Mason 1994, 136).

The continuing power of blood in the definition of a fit parent was also evident in some of the most publicized and heart-wrenching custody disputes of the era. Most notorious was the Baby Jessica case, in which the courts struggled between giving custody of a young girl to her birth parents or to the foster parents she had known since infancy. In awarding custody, the court focused on whether the parental rights of the biological father had been correctly terminated. As Nelkin and Lindee make clear, the decision to take the child from the family that raised her and return the girl to her biological parents not only provoked public outrage but also revealed the continuing tension between definitions of fit parents based on social parenting and biology (Nelkin and Lindee 1995).

Such cases led Skolnick to conclude, "Many commentators, though, believe that the child's best interests are in fact served by growing up with biological parents, and that parents not only have a right to their children but that 'natural bonds of affection' lead parents to care for their children in a way that no 'stranger' could" (Skolnick 1998, 239). She maintains that in "recent years, the traditional biological concept of family in American culture and law has been joined by what might be called a new biologicalism, a growing sense that the true essence of a person is rooted in the primordial differences of gender, race, ethnicity, genes. It's true that the recent advances in genetic research have made biological information about one's family background an important part of a person's medical history. But the new biologicalism is a much broader cultural phenomenon that encompasses identity politics and the emphasis on ethnic roots, the search movement among adoptees, and the anti-adoption movement that has emerged in recent years" (240). And she concludes, for "a variety of reasons, then, the facts of biological parenthood carry more legal weight than in the past. Courts have shown a strong preference for awarding custody to what they call 'natural parents' whether or not a parent-child relationship exists. Large numbers of adults who have actually nurtured and raised children—relatives, stepparents, and foster parents—have no legal standing" (242).

Custody law changes since the mid twentieth century reveal the continued expansion of the legal definition of a fit parent, but also that it is a trend leavened by the persistent power of blood ties. The expanding notion of fit parent based on social parenting certainly lent credence to the contention by Nelkin and Lindee that "actual family units are sustained, however, more by social forces than biological realities. Many professionals define the family as a social unit that may include relationships based on emotional connection and commitment rather than on biological ties" (Nelkin and Lindee 1995, 77). And such a conviction clearly expresses the historical reality that fit parenthood is an evolving idea based on changing notions of proper parental roles and duties defined in terms of child nurture. However, even though parenthood has become less equated with biology, clashes between social and biological dimensions of parenting continue, as disputes about the custodial rights of foster and stepparents amply reveal. The belief that the claims of blood take precedence still resonates strongly in American society and raises questions about the significance of nurture as an exception to the blood rule. The demise of maternal preference makes such uncertainties critical as public officials and private families confront new challenges such as DNA testing.

Paternal Responsibility

The redefinition of fit parents, and particularly the linked decline of maternal preference and rise of paternal custody rights, points to a basic reconceptualization of paternal responsibility in the second half of the twentieth century. The demise of the nineteenth-century family law regime stemmed in part from new ideas of gender roles that revised the place of fathers in the American home. Attempts by some fathers to claim a more active role as child rearers ignited debate on men's parenting potential. A fathers' rights movement emerged to champion paternal prerogatives, as was evident in the strident declaration of breadwinning grievances by Jon Conine in his 1989 polemic *Father's Rights*: "Society cannot take away a father's rights to his children and expect him to cheerfully pay child support. Society cannot expect a father to make enough money to support two separate households. Society cannot afford to support mothers who choose not to work" (2). Such pronouncements help explain why the parental possibilities of fathers became contested in ways they had not been since the rise of the modern family in the late eighteenth century.

However, demands for greater paternal rights were buffeted by contradictory trends, much as in the contemporary debates about parental fitness. A new sense of the importance of fathering and fathers was leavened by a declining presence of fathers in homes as the divorce rate soared, along with charges that more deadbeat dads were failing to pay child support. Simultaneously, the sexual revolution severed the link between marriage and parenthood to further complicate the parental claims of men. And even though the nurturing capabilities of men underwent a reexamination, breadwinning remained the primary component of paternal responsibility and the nurturing commitments of most fathers remained suspect. In fact, the "dominant form of fatherhood . . . is one of abandonment or lack of connection" (Dowd 2000, 35, 37). Thus, despite the changes of the era, questions and questioning about fathers as nurturing parents continued as they had since the birth of the modern family.

The conflicting concerns about paternal custody claims became evident in disputes about the custodial rights of unwed fathers. In the 1960s, courts began to grant custodial rights to unwed fathers in addition to their traditional obligation of support. They did so amid rising rates of illegitimate births and broad questioning of the very utility of illegitimacy as social policy, as well as the persistent concern about punishing innocent children for parental sin that had dominated the debate on illegitimacy since the 1780s (Woodhouse 2000).

Against this background, the U.S. Supreme Court remade the custodial rights of unwed fathers in the 1972 case of *Stanley v. Illinois*. Peter Stanley challenged an Illinois statute that made children wards of the court on the death of the mother. He claimed that equal protection under the Constitution required that he be treated like married fathers, who were presumed fit custodians under Illinois law whether they were divorced, separated, or widowed. The Supreme Court agreed, and determined that there must be a fitness hearing to determine custody, as there would be for all natural parents in such circumstances. Justice Byron White maintained that the "private interests here: that of a man in the children that he has sired and raised, undeniably warrants deference and, absent a powerful countervailing interest, protection."

However, judges continued to look on the custody claims of unwed fathers with suspicion. They demanded evidence of a parental commitment from men like Stanley and in doing so used social parenting as the gauge for judging paternal responsibility. The Supreme Court explained the new approach in the 1983 case of *Lehr v. Robertson*. The justices rejected the adoption challenge of a man who had never lived with his daughter. Casting aside his plea that he was denied equal protection under the Constitution because, as an unwed father, he had received no notice or opportunity to protest termination of his parental rights, the majority of the Supreme Court agreed with Justice John Paul Stevens that "the significance of the biological connection is that it offers the natural father an opportunity that no other male possesses to develop a relationship with his offspring. If he grasps that opportunity and accepts some measure of responsibility for the child's future, he may enjoy the blessings of the parent-child relationship and make uniquely valuable contributions to the child's development. If he fails to do so, the Federal Constitution will not automatically compel a State to listen to his opinion of where the child's best interests lie."

A decision of this type meant that unwed fathers who demonstrated a willingness to act as parents could secure rights to visitation, consent to adoption, and inheritance, which would have been unthinkable under the previous family law regime. That reality led Leslie Harris to worry that "under the statutes and case law of many states, custodial claims of unwed fathers are protected to a far greater extent than the Supreme Court has said is constitutionally necessary, even when this protection comes at the price of disrupting functional, but not biologically related, families" (Harris 1996, 468). The consequence, she maintains, is that as "the importance of marriage for determining legal father-hood has declined, the law has developed to give relatively little protection or responsibility to men who take on parental responsibilities to provide for and nurture children to whom they are not biologically connected" (473).

And yet unwed fathers did not secure rights as extensive as those of their married peers. The Court narrowed but retained the law's long-standing commitment to matrimony by limiting the rights of these men. Moreover, as in the past, public authorities remained more concerned with ensuring that at least one parent supported the child than with considerations for the child's best interests. These realities meant that unwed fathers remained suspect parents whose custody rights were tied to the fulfillment of paternal responsibility, and expressed the conviction that fatherhood entailed more than biological connections. In fact, legal scholar Dorothy Roberts argues that "recent Supreme Court opinions involving parental rights of unwed fathers suggest that legal paternity continues to depend more on the father's relationship with his children's mother than on a genetic tie with the children" (Roberts 1995, 253). And because, unlike Peter Stanley, most unwed fathers did not live with their offspring and had little or no contact with them, those rights remained limited. In this way, the changing custody rights of unwed fathers underscored the reality that legal authorities continued to act on the assumption that legal parentage arises more fundamentally from female than male biology. A mother's biological connection to her child imposes an automatic social relationship, whereas fathers remain freer to choose whether to develop a social tie or not. Thus the law still viewed fathers' social relationship to their children as more of a chosen, cultural creation than an inevitable product of their genetic tie to their offspring. The changing legal rights of unwed fathers continued another fundamental reality embedded in the legal conception of paternal responsibility and expressed in revealing language by family law scholar Karen Czapanskiy (1991), who reminds us that mothers are parental draftees while men are volunteers.

Changing views of paternal rights and duties combined with the increased resort to divorce and the advent of DNA testing to ignite a new debate about the traditional presumption that children born within marriage are fathered by the husband. As more men like Gerald Miscovich used genetic tests to file legal claims as duped dads, the conflicts embedded in the marital presumption between male victimization by adulterous wives and children's interests in maintaining established relationships could no longer be avoided. The new scientific precision made possible with DNA testing forced a reevaluation of the traditional rule. It had to be defended with new arguments or discarded as outmoded morally as well as technologically (Glennon 2000). The resulting debate has focused on the tension between social parenting and biological responsibility that strikes at the heart of cultural notions of fatherhood and thus paternal responsibility.

Challenges to the presumption such as that made by Miscovich have produced legal confusion and contradictory decisions. Generally, courts have refused to hold husbands responsible for other men's offspring and so have sanctioned discarding these children. As Glennon summarizes the situation, "Most courts have found that acceptance of the paternal role and provision of support during the marriage does not create reliance or detriment. They have differed about both the existence and importance of emotional or financial harm to affected children" (Glennon 2000, 579–80). And although all states continue to recognize a marital presumption of paternity, few continue to treat the presumption as irrebuttable or they strictly limit the circumstances in which it can be rebutted. Thirty-three states now permit a man claiming to be the biological father to rebut the marital presumption. However, uncertainty persists about whether men should be able to rebut the marital presumption of paternity through genetic testing. As in the past, it springs from doubt about whether biology should be the fundamental basis for parental rights.

The complexities of the renewed debate on the legitimacy and efficacy of the marital presumption arose in their most dramatic fashion in what would become the iconic case in modern debates about paternal responsibility: *Michael H. v. Gerald D.* (1989), a U.S. Supreme Court decision involving California's marital presumption. Blood tests established the paternity of a neighbor, Michael, and the mother and daughter lived with him at various times but eventually returned to the husband, Gerald. Denied visitation privileges, Michael filed an action to establish his paternity and thus a right to visitation. Even though a court-appointed psychologist recommended that the mother retain sole custody but Michael be allowed continued contact, the state courts ruled that, under the California statute, the biological father lacked standing to challenge the marital presumption. A divided Supreme Court upheld the California ruling allowing the mother and her husband to block the biological father from asserting parental rights. The plurality opinion by Justice Antonin Scalia invoked nature to rule out a compromise allowing for multiple fatherhood: "California law, like nature itself, makes no provision for dual fatherhood." He interpreted the due process clause as a protection against unnecessary and unwanted changes, which in this case meant preventing "future generations from lightly casting aside important traditional values." To illustrate the horrors that might arise from linking fathers' rights to biological ties in a way that undermined established families, Justice Scalia used the example of a child born of a rape. In dissent, Justice Brennan countered, "In the plurality's constitutional universe, we may not take notice of the fact that the original reasons for the conclusive presumption of paternity are out of place in a world in which blood tests can prove virtually beyond a shadow of a doubt who sired a particular child and in which the fact of illegitimacy no longer plays the burdensome and stigmatizing role it once did." He complained that the challenged statute insisted on labeling Gerald the father "in the face of evidence showing a 98 percent probability that her father is Michael."

The case sparked intense debates. Professor Barbara Woodhouse argued that it "illustrates the effects of the Court's historic focus on the rights of parents to custody, rather than on reciprocal rights in intimate family relationships shared by both parent and child" (Woodhouse 2000, 431). Another family law scholar, Diane S. Kaplan, contended that continued reliance on the presumption ignited a clash between legal truth and scientific truth: "When a legal presumption is no longer consistent with the social values that previously justified its use, the presumption becomes simultaneously both true and false. The incongruity between law and science invites conflict rather than constancy as the presumption obscures rather than answers the questions it was created to resolve: What is a father? Is fatherhood a biological question or a socio-legal construct? Should courts uphold legal constructs that conflict with scientific facts that may be highly disruptive of our social order?" (Kaplan 2000, 73).

Despite the debates on the newly recognized custody rights of some fathers and the continued legitimacy of the presumption of paternity, breadwinning remained at the core of the legal definition of paternal responsibility. And securing child support remained a critical if not growing problem, in part because the singular focus on finding deadbeat dads highlighted the persistent pattern of male evasion that has dominated experiences of enforced paternal responsibility. Thus attorney Laura M. Morgan reports that "65 per cent of absent fathers contribute no child support or alimony and only 5.5 per cent of absent fathers contribute as much as $5,000 per year, while 91 per cent of married fathers contribute earnings of at least $5,000 to the total family income" (Morgan 1999, 710). The persistence of the breadwinning role and of the determination of the public and state authorities to hold men financially accountable for their offspring has buttressed the reliance on blood ties as the primary basis for fatherhood, as well as its converse: no blood ties, no responsibility. This logic remains persuasive, Harris explains, because "the argument that a man who is responsible for a child's conception should be responsible for the child's support because he has voluntarily undertaken this obligation has a strong appeal, especially in a society that such as ours regards voluntary assumption as an obvious justification for imposing legal duties" (Harris 1996, 473). There has been no second-guessing, no questioning about this paternal responsibility, only a determined quest for greater effectiveness.

The most significant changes in support policies have been the growing role of the federal government in erecting a national system for securing child support and the increased reliance on DNA testing to determine paternity. Federal acts enabled state child support programs to acquire a vast array of enforcement remedies, such as the attachment of income tax refunds, bank accounts, property, and other assets. As a result, case-by-case procedures for seizing and attaching the income and assets of delinquent nonresidential parents were replaced with streamlined, automatic, administrative, and computer-driven processes. They also mandated the use of DNA testing. Statutory reforms and technological innovations led to a great wave of paternity filings in the late 1990s. Thousands of men became legal fathers with attendant rights and child support responsibilities. Critically, genetic testing for paternity came to be seen as a magic bullet for state budgets, with the unintended consequence of heightening the tension between social parenting and paternal responsibility. And, as in the past, paternity hearings remained wedded to the assumption that biological fatherhood was the fundamental basis for paternal financial responsibility for a child, and the child support system continued to focus on the correct identification of the biological father. The question of whether a social parent-child relationship had been established was thus made fundamentally irrelevant (Pearson 2000).

The rising divorce rate also produced a bumper crop of deadbeat dads. Concern about the support consequences of migratory divorce in the 1940s and 1950s led states to adopt a model law (nicknamed the Skipping Pappy Act) designed to pursue a nonpaying former spouse across state lines. Yet the effort to compel financial support proved ineffective, and the disengagement of most fathers from children after divorce continued unabated. Breadwinning and evasion clashed in cases involving male responsibilities to children who were not living with them while also reinforcing the link of paternal rights with blood ties (Mason 1994; Harris 1996).

The dramatic changes in family law and in households during the second half of the twentieth century and into the twenty-first have significantly altered both the definitions of fit parents and the nature of paternal responsibility. The social ideal of fit parents continued to expand as social parenting proved to be a consistently appealing and expansive concept. However, biology not only remained a critical component of legal definitions of fit parents, it may well have increased in significance. At the same time, men gained new household rights and roles, as paternal responsibility, too, became a more expansive concept. Yet breadwinning, resistance to child support responsibilities, and fear of unwanted and unfairly imposed paternity remained central to men's family practices. As a result, DNA testing exposed the conflicts, contradictions, and fissures of the American family order.

Conclusion

Like many excursions into the past, this one has produced a cautionary tale. Problems in the present, even those caused by seemingly radical new technology, have a past. That past is complicated, even contradictory, yet critical. It does not dictate present policy but helps us more clearly understand the choices that must be made. In terms of creating guidelines for the use of DNA testing in child custody cases, it is a history that centers on the development of fit parents and paternal responsibility in the law of child custody. And it is a history that produces not a single message but clashing messages. New legal definitions of fit parents that emerged with the advent of the modern family led to the creation and then development of social parenting as a fundamental standard for judging child rearers. Social parenting became an expansive concept based on the primacy of nurture in defining the best interests of the young. The conviction that the best custodian of the young should be defined in terms of nurture diminished the power of blood ties as the only legitimate basis for custodial claims. By contrast, the development of paternal responsibility has focused on the male household roles, particularly breadwinning, that highlight blood ties, fiscal duties, and evasion. It has strengthened male resistance to unwanted fatherhood and promoted the belief that men should be responsible only for children related to them by blood. Legal rules about fit parents and paternal responsibility are thus historically conditioned ideals embedded in American law and society. And, most critically, the persistent tensions and problems between the laws governing fit parents and parental responsibility helped ensure that the response to DNA testing in child custody cases would be framed as a clash between children's needs and father's rights, between duped dads and discarded children.

And yet trying to give DNA testing a past also tells us that this clash does not produce an inevitable result. Quite the contrary: the history of both concepts—parental fitness and parental responsibility—underscores only that choices have been made in the past and will be made in the present. And it tells us that those decisions will entail sacrifices and will have real and long-lasting consequences in people's lives. The basic question suggested by the past is whether that sacrifice will be made by adults or children. The former choice—making social parenting the basis for the use of information from DNA tests in child custody cases—would mean making the nurturing needs of the young the primary consideration. In its own way this would be a radical innovation in the law, but one with some legal antecedents, as this chapter has suggested. The latter choice—enforcing paternal responsibility despite a tradition of evasion and legitimation—would also be a radical act. It could occur only with a new sense of male responsibility and parental voluntarism. As Leslie Harris argues,

> We need, instead, rules that directly encourage and reward adults' caretaking behavior. Such an approach is, however, threatening. It would not affect children who live throughout their childhoods with their married biological parents or children living with adults who have devised such arrangements on their own. However, it would change the lives of families struggling to integrate new relationships with the remnants of old ones. It would challenge our collective assumptions about the origins of responsibility and even what being responsible means. We must be willing to face these challenges, though, for equating biological and legal parentage disserves the interests of many children (Harris 1996, 485).

Though the past does not tell us which choice will be made, it does suggest that transformative change is possible. It has occurred in history; it can happen now, even in such fundamental institutions as the family. If people are willing to make transformative choices, then change is possible. But fathers and children must want it. Recounting the history of fit parents and paternal responsibility in an attempt to give DNA testing in child custody cases a past allows us to understand the current realities of children in America in a new and, I hope, liberating way, one that frees us to tackle the present with historically chastened understanding and yet also with renewed hope.

BIBLIOGRAPHY

Adoption of Galen. 1997. 680 N.E.2d 70, 73 (Mass.).

Adoption of Tammy. 1993. 610 N.E.2d 315 (Mass.).

Appell, A. R. 2001. Virtual mothers and the meaning of parenthood. *University of Michigan Journal of Law Reform* 334:728–32.

Bartholet, E. 1999. *Family Bonds, Adoption, Infertility, and the New World of Child Production.* Boston: Beacon Press.

Basch, N. 1999. *Framing American Divorce from the Revolutionary Generation to the Victorians.* Berkeley and Los Angeles: University of California Press.

Beils v. Furbish. 1855. 39 Me. 469 (Me.).

Brinig, M. F., C. E. Schneider, and L. E. Teitelbaum. 1999. *Family Law in Action—A Reader.* Dayton, OH: Anderson.

Burgee, R. 1956. The Lord Mansfield rule and the presumption of legitimacy. *Maryland Law Review* 16:236–44.

Caban v. Mohammed. 1979. 441 U.S. 380.

Carp, E. W. 1998. *Family Matters, Secrecy and Disclosure in the History of Adoption,* chap. 1. Cambridge: Harvard University Press.

Chambers, D. L., and M. S. Wald, 1985. Part III, *Smith v. OFFER.* In *In the Interest of Children, Advocacy, Law Reform, and Public Policy,* ed. R. H. Mnookin, 67–147. New York: W. H. Freeman.

Chapsky v. Wood. 1881. 26 Kan. 650, 653 (Kan.).

Chused, R. H. 1994. *Private Acts in Public Places: A Social History of Divorce in the Formative Era of American Family Law.* Philadelphia: University of Pennsylvania Press.

Clark v. Bradstreet. 1888. 15 A. 56 (Me.).

Conine, J. 1989. *Father's Rights: The Sourcebook for Dealing with Child Support.* New York: Walker.

Cott, N. F. 2000. *Public Vows: A History of Marriage and the Nation.* Cambridge: Harvard University Press.

Cross v. Cross. 1831. 3 Paige 139, 140 (N.Y.).

Czapanskiy, K. 1991. Volunteers and draftees: The struggle for parental equality. *UCLA Law Review* 38:1415–81.

Davis v. Salisbury. 1804. 1 Root 278 (Conn.).

Doering, C. 1925–26. Evidence: Admissibility of evidence of resemblance where paternity is in issue. *Central Law Quarterly* 11:380–85.

Dolgin, J. L. 2000. Choice, tradition, and the new genetics. *Connecticut Law Review* 32: 527–34.

Dowd, N. 2000. *Redefining Fatherhood.* New York: New York University Press.

Dubois v. Johnson. 1884. 96 Ind. 6 (Ind.).

Dye v. Geiger. 1996. 554 N.W.2d 538 (Iowa).

Ex parte Crouse. 1839. 4 Whart. 9, 11–12 (Pa.).

Gilmantown v. Ham. 1859. 39 N.H. 108, 112–13 (N.H.).

Glennon, T. 2000. Somebody's child: Evaluating the erosion of the marital presumption of paternity. *West Virginia Law Review* 102:555–59.

Goodrich v. Goodrich. 1870. 44 Ala. 670 (Ala.).

Green v. Campbell. 1891. 35 W.Va. 699 (W.Va.).

Griswold, R. 1993. *Fatherhood in America: A History.* New York: Basic Books.

Grossberg, M. 1985. *Governing the Hearth: Law and the Family in Nineteenth Century America,* chap. 7. Chapel Hill: University of North Carolina Press.

———. 1995. *A Judgment for Solomon: The d'Hauteville Case and Legal Experience in Antebellum America.* New York: Cambridge University Press.

———. 1999. Citizens and families: A Jeffersonian vision of domestic relations and generational change. In *Thomas Jefferson and the Education of a Citizen,* ed. J. Gilbreath, 3–27. Washington, DC: Library of Congress.

———. 2000. How to give the present a past? Family law in the United States 1950–2000. In *Cross Currents, Family Law and Policy in the United States and England,* ed. S. N. Katz, J. Eekelaar, and M. Maclean, 1–29. Oxford: Oxford University Press.

Halem, L. C. 1980. *Divorce Reform: Changing Legal and Social Perspectives.* New York: Free Press.

Harris, L. J. 1996. Reconsidering the criteria for legal fatherhood. *Utah Law Review* 1996:461–85.

Hartog, H. 2000. *Man and Wife in America: A History,* chaps 1–4. Cambridge: Harvard University Press.

Hitchcock v. Grant. 1789. 1 Root 107 (Conn.).

Howe, R. A. W. 2000. Parenthood in the United States. In *Cross Currents, Family Law and Policy in the United States and England,* ed. S. N. Katz, J. Eekelaar, and M. Maclean, 206–7. Oxford: Oxford University Press.

Hudson v. Hills. 1836. 8 N.H. 417, 418 (N.H.).

In re Vance. 1891. 92 Cal. 195 (Cal.).

In the Matter of Mitchell. 1836. 1 Charlton 489–95 (Ga.).

Jacobs v. Pollard. 1852. 10 Cush. 284 (Mass.)

Kaplan, D. S. 2000. Comparative comment: Why truth is not a defense in paternity actions. *Texas Journal of Women and the Law* 10:69–81.

Kent, J. 1826. *Commentaries on American Law,* 2:211–12. New York: O. Halsted.

Kimmel, M. 1997. *Manhood in America: A Cultural History.* New York: Free Press.

Lehr v. Robertson. 1983. 463 U.S. 248, 262.

Lewin, T. 2001. In genetic testing for paternity, law often lags behind science. *New York Times,* 11 March.

Mahoney, W. 1994. *Stepfamilies and the Law.* Ann Arbor: University of Michigan Press.

Mason, M. A. 1994. *From Father's Property to Children's Rights: The History of Child Custody in the United States,* chap. 2. New York: Columbia University Press.

May, M. 1988. The "problem of duty": Family desertion in the progressive era. *Social Service Review* 62:40–60.

Michael H. v. Gerald D. 1989. 491 U.S. 110, 113–16, 128–30.

Michigan Law Review. 1930. Note: The Lord Mansfield rule as to bastardizing the issue. 3:79–87.

Milburn v. Milburn. 1923. 254 S.W. 121 (Tex.).

Mintz, S., and S. Kellogg. 1988. *Domestic Revolutions: A Social History of American Family Life.* New York: Free Press.

Miscovich v. Miscovich. 1997. 688 A.2d. 726 (Pa. Super. 1997); *aff'd,* 720 A.2d 764 (Pa. 1998), *cert. denied,* 526 U.S. 1113 (1999).

Morgan, L. M. 1999. Family law in 2000: Private and public support of the family: From welfare state to poor laws. *Family Law Quarterly* 33:705–18.

Nelkin, D., and M. S. Lindee. 1995. *DNA Mystique: The Gene as Cultural Icon.* New York: W. H. Freeman.

O'Donovan, K. 1988. A right to know one's parentage. *International Journal of Law and the Family* 2:31–33.

Pearson, J. 2000. A forum for every fuss: The growth of court services and ADR treatment for family law cases in the United States. In *Cross Currents, Family Law and Policy in the United States and England,* ed. S. N. Katz, J. Eekelaar, and M. Maclean, 513–31. Oxford: Oxford University Press.

People v. Hickey. 1899. 86 Ill. App. 20 (Ill. Ct. App.).

Phillips, R. 1988. *Putting Asunder: A History of Divorce in Western Society,* chaps. 11, 12. New York: Cambridge University Press.

Quillion v. Walcott. 1978. 434 U.S. 246.

Report of the D'Hauteville Case. 1840. Philadelphia: William S. Martien.

Roberts, D. 1995. The genetic tie. *University of Chicago Law Review* 62:253–55.

Rotundo, A. E. 1993. *American Manhood: Transformations in Masculinity from the Revolution to the Modern Era,* chaps. 1–7. New York: Basic Books.

R.R. v. J.M. 1825. 3 N.H. 135 (N.H.).

Schnooner v. Commonwealth. 1809. Litt. Sel. Cas. 88, 90–91 (Ky.).

Schouler, J. 1906. *A Treatise on the Law of Domestic Relations,* 6th ed., 2:2034–35. Boston: Little, Brown.

Scoggins v. Scoggins. 1879. 80 N.C. 318 (N.C.).

Shapiro, E. D., S. Reifler, and C. L. Psome. 1992–93. The DNA paternity test: Legislating the future paternity action. *Journal of Law and Health* 7:16–19.

Skolnick, A. 1998. Solomon's children: The new biologism, psychological parenthood, attachment theory, and the best interest standard. In *All Our Families: New Policies for a New Century,* ed. M. A. Mason, A. Skolnick, and S. D. Sugarman, 236–55. New York: Oxford University Press.

Smith v. Organization of Foster Families for Equality and Reform. 1977. 431 U.S. 816, 843.

Stanley v. Illinois. 1972. 405 U.S. 645, 658, 651.

State v. Bowles. 1860. 7 Jones 579 (N.C.).

State v. Goode. 1849. 10 Ire. 49, 51–52 (N.C.).

State v. Lee. 1847. 7 Ire. 265 (N.C.).

State v. Waller. 1913. 90 Kan. 829.

Stiles v. Eastman. 1828. 21 Pick. 132 (Mass.).

Stones v. Keeling. 1804. 5 Call 143, 146–47 (Va.).

Strasser, M. 1997. *Legally Wed: Same-Sex Marriage and the Constitution.* Ithaca, NY: Cornell University Press.

Swift, Z. 1795. *A System of Laws and the State of Connecticut,* 208. New Haven: S. Converse.

Umlauf v. Umlauf. 1888. 27 Ill. App. 275 (Ill. Ct. App.).

Wand v. Wand. 1860. 14 Cal. 512 (Cal.).

Washaw v. Gimble. 1887. 59 Ark. 351 (Ark.).

Wigmore, J. 1904. *A Treatise on the Law of Evidence,* 3 vols. Chicago.

Willrich, M. 2000. Home slackers: Men, the state, and welfare in modern America. *Journal of American History* 87:460–69.

Woodhouse, B. 2000. The status of children: A story of emerging rights. In *Cross Currents, Family Law and Policy in the United States and England,* ed. S. N. Katz, J. Eekelaar, and M. Maclean, 430–31. Oxford: Oxford University Press.

Wright v. Hicks. 1854. 15 Ga. 160.

Zainaldin, J. 1979. The emergence of a modern American family law: Child custody, adoption, and the courts, 1776–1851. *Northwestern University Law Review* 73:1038–89.

CHAPTER EIGHT

Guiding Principles for Picking Parents

Elizabeth Bartholet, J.D.

We live in an era in which DNA testing can provide definitive proof as to whether a genetic link exists between an adult and a child where, until recently, such proof was not possible. We need to decide whether this means that the law should place greater emphasis on biology in defining parentage than it previously has. I title this chapter "Guiding Principles for Picking Parents" to emphasize the societal choice inherent in all decisions about parentage. Despite the frequent talk of DNA "parentage testing," I deny that this kind of testing, whatever it may be called by its proponents, is truly parentage testing. DNA tests can determine whether there is a genetic link between two people—whether a given man's sperm helped create a given child—but not whether that man is or is not that child's *parent*. In fact, biology has never been all-determinative in defining parentage, whether in nature or under law. In nature some animals are raised by both biological parents, but in most species "fathers" exist only in the sense that they create life (Popenoe 1994). Further, like humans, animals sometimes "adopt" others' offspring.

For as long as law has governed various family matters among humans, it has looked at biology as only one among a number of factors to be used in deciding how to allocate parental rights and responsibilities. Given that society will, through law, decide on *some* parent-picking principles, we need to think what those principles should be. We want principles that will work for the larger society, which means principles that will work for children so that they grow up healthy, happy, and able to function as adults to make that society work.

Today, many men who have been functioning as social fathers are in a position to discover that they are not biological fathers. Some of them are demanding, often in the context of divorce, to be released from their parental responsibilities. This is not a small problem: recent studies show that surprisingly high percentages of children born in the context of marriage or marriage-like relationships are not genetically related to their mothers' partners, the men who have been functioning as their fathers (Anderlik and Rothstein 2002, 221–24; Welstead 2003, 151–52). It seems beyond obvious that, if we really care about children, we should give them the permanent parenting that generations of child psychiatrists and child welfare specialists have told us that children need. Once a child-parent relationship has been created, we should not let it be destroyed simply because there is no DNA match. Parenting, once undertaken, is or should be a lifetime responsibility.

However, not all courts and legislatures find this obvious. Many are releasing men who have established parenting relationships from any parental responsibilities on the basis of DNA testing or similarly definitive proof that they have no genetic link to the children at issue (Roberts 2004; Anderlik and Rothstein 2002, 225–27). For example, an appeals court in Pennsylvania recently ruled that it was appropriate to release a man from his parental support obligations for a child he had fathered for eleven years, from the time of her birth during his marriage to the mother, through several years of marriage, and through the years after his divorce until DNA testing revealed he was not the genetic father. At that point, as the trial court tolerantly put it, he "as gently as possible removed himself from the child's life in a way that he felt would cause the child the least amount of anguish and hurt" (*Doran v. Doran* 2003) and moved to terminate support. Comparable cases abound. Likewise, some state legislatures have passed, and others are considering, laws that would as a general matter release men from parental responsibilities based on proof that they are not the genetic fathers (Roberts 2004; Anderlik and Rothstein 2002). The fathers' rights movement has been active in promoting these judicial and legislative developments.

Many of our societal rules for defining parentage were developed in an era when children were ordinarily the genetic product of the husband and wife who raised them, and, in any event, it was difficult to establish that they were not. The world has changed. We now have DNA tests that can easily and conclusively establish whether there is any genetic link between parent and child. We now have a significant breakdown in the nuclear family, with men and women moving with far greater freedom in and out of different marital and marital-like relationships, same-sex as well as opposite-sex, and with children more often being raised at least in part by stepparents or stepparent equivalents. We now have reproductive technologies that enable the use of third parties' eggs, sperm, gestational services, and embryos to produce children to be raised by parents who may have no genetic or biological connection to them. This newly available DNA information, these newly complex family arrangements, and these new reproductive technologies have together produced a raft of new questions about how to define parentage.

In this chapter I provide some guiding principles for picking parents in this new era. While I do not get into the specifics of designing model legislation or analyzing individual hard cases, my hope is that these principles will prove useful to those enterprises.

Core Principles

Law Governs

Law decides who is and who is not a parent and whether and on what basis someone who is a parent is allowed to stop being one. Today, some talk as if something they might call "natural law" governed—as if, once you know the DNA, you know who is and who is not the parent. The highest court in Massachusetts recently decided in *In re Paternity of Cheryl* (2001) that a man who had functioned as a social and support father for six years would continue to be responsible for child support even after DNA testing revealed that he was not the genetic father. On talk shows I found myself defending the court's decision against attack by men who shouted at me that it was unfair to make this "nonfather" pay child support. They did not want to hear me explain that the court had decided that in fact he *was* the father, by virtue of the extended parenting relationship, regardless of whether he was genetically linked to the child. In our system the law decides who is a parent.

It is true that law has traditionally accorded significant weight to biology in defining parentage. For example, the law assigns those who give birth presumptive rights to parent their progeny. It is also true that in a few cases the U.S. Supreme Court has spoken in natural law terms, citing fundamental prelaw human rights, in upholding genetic parents' rights as protected under the federal Constitution. These cases seemed to put some limits on the degree to which states can deny parenting rights to people who have a combination of biology and social relationship on their side. However, in a more recent case,

Michael H. v. Gerald D. (1989), the Supreme Court upheld a California law that defined a sperm father who had a significant social parenting relationship with his progeny as a nonfather, and defined the husband of the child's mother as the legal father. So today's Court has signaled its willingness to provide the states with significant leeway to determine who is a parent and how prominently biology should figure in that determination.

Parenting law has often defined as parents persons who have no biological link to the child in preference to those who have such a link. Traditionally, state law has defined a husband as parent of the children born to his wife during the marriage, regardless of any evidence indicating that another man was actually the sperm father (Anderlik and Rothstein 2002). This was the kind of law upheld as constitutional in the *Michael H.* case noted above. Adoption law defines as full legal parents persons who have no biological link to the child. For decades, state law has defined a husband as the father of children his wife produces using sperm from another man through artificial insemination (Anderlik and Rothstein 2002).

The dominant trend in current law is in the direction of reducing the importance of biology as a factor in defining parentage (Carbone and Cahn 2003, 1020). Increasing emphasis is being placed on established and intended parenting relationships, with these factors sometimes weighing equally with or even outweighing biology. Law has focused increasingly on *established* parenting relationships in part to deal with the new complexity of family life, as the nuclear family has broken up and children are more often dependent on nurturing relationships with people other than their genetic parents. Both courts and legislatures have helped develop the functional parent doctrine, giving those who have developed parenting relationships with children the right to come into court and compete with those who became parents through biology for some piece of the total parenting rights package.

Some courts have held that those who have functioned as unmarried co-parents with biological parents have developed true parenting rights by virtue of their de facto parenting and are entitled at the point of "divorce" to fight for visitation and even for primary custody. Some legislatures have given persons traditionally treated as nonparents the right to come into court to ask for visitation rights based on some prior relationship with the child that would make visitation consistent with the child's best interests. Although the U.S. Supreme Court struck down one such law in the recent *Troxel v. Granville* (2000), that case involved a "breathtakingly broad" statute that gave rights to people who had not established a functional parent relationship. The parties asking for visitation rights in the case were grandparents who claimed only a classic grandparenting relationship. *Troxel* makes it clear that "parents" are constitutionally protected against inappropriate intervention in their families by nonparents, but it does nothing to limit how states may define parents and thus does little to limit development of the functional parent trend. The influential American Law Institute gave important backing to the functional parent doctrine in its 2002 *Principles of the Law of Family Dissolution*. These principles create two new classes of parent, parents by estoppel and de facto parents, according nonbiological parents who have functioned as parents varying degrees of parental status.

Intended parenting is also an increasingly important determinant of parentage, as reproductive technology multiplies the number of people involved in producing a child (Bartholet 1999a). Those who want to parent but cannot produce a child with their own bodies have more and more options in today's world. They can look to others for genetic material—sperm, eggs, and embryos—and for pregnancy and birthing services. They generally use the private law of contract to make deals with the providers of these goods and services in an attempt to guarantee that they, the intended parents, are recognized in the end as the actual parents. Although there are few guarantees that these contracts will be honored by the courts if it comes to a legal battle, for the most part people do honor their contracts and intent wins out. Thus, for example, only a tiny percentage of the birth mothers involved in surrogacy arrangements change their minds after birth and decide to keep their child, even though it is extremely unlikely that their contracts to surrender the child would be specifically enforced by the courts.

Public law has generally not interfered in these contractual arrangements to insist that biology should trump intent. Indeed, public law seems to be moving in the direction, albeit slowly, of ensuring that intent will govern and that these arrangements whereby people agree that children should be spun off by their biological creators to be raised by others are legitimate. In the adoption world, universally applicable public law forbids the use of money to persuade birth parents to surrender their progeny for others to raise, largely in deference to the importance of biology as a parent-defining factor. Screening of adoptive parents for parental fitness is required to address concerns about the parenting capacity of unrelated parents. But in the world of reproductive technology, there is almost no public law that requires fitness screening for genetically unrelated parents or forbids the sale of genetic material, pregnancy services, or, after the baby's birth, parental rights. There could be few stronger social statements as to the *un*importance of biology to parenting in this modern world of child production.

From the perspective of the intending parents, biology is of course extremely important in terms of what drives the various practices of assisted reproductive technology. Those buying sperm, eggs, and embryos often do so in the hope that at least one of the two intended parents will have a genetic or at least a gestational connection to the future child. Even without such connection, the intended parents tend to search for genetic contributors who will produce a child that looks a lot like the child those parents might have produced with their own genes. But, in the end, intended parents are to a great degree settling for biologically unrelated parenthood. Moreover, from the perspective of social policy making, our law's failure to regulate reproductive technology in the way it regulates adoption indicates, at a minimum, significant societal ambivalence about the relevance of biology to parenting.

Biology: Only a Factor

The background debate. As discussed above, U.S. law treats biology as only one factor relevant to defining parentage, and as one of increasingly limited relevance. However, the fact that science today gives us new possibilities for determining who is and who is not biologically related has provided new energy for those who think biology *should* be determinative. We *can* figure out who produced the child biologically, therefore we *should* declare those persons the parents and all others the nonparents—so goes the thinking of these new geneticists.

We need to figure out just how important biology should be in determining parentage. We need to address the demands made by the men who are running into court waving their DNA test results to demand that they be relieved of parenting responsibilities. And we need to address the growing schism between the realm of traditional family law, which makes biology extremely important in defining parentage, even if not always determinative, and the realm of reproductive technology, which treats biology as quite unimportant.

My own view is that biology is clearly not *all*-important, as the new geneticists claim, nor is it *as* important as traditional family law makes it. I have critiqued elsewhere the claims made by many in the adoption world that genetics should be seen as central to parenting, claims that children raised by nonbiological parents are doomed to suffer genealogical bewilderment and that birth parents deprived of the opportunity to raise their birth children are doomed to suffer forever from the breach in genetic continuity (Bartholet 1999a, 51–61). Such claims rely on little other than psychological theorizing, together with junk science. Empirical studies show that children fare just as well when raised by adoptive parents as when raised by birth parents, as long as they are placed in infancy so that they have one set of nurturing parents from early on (164–86). I have also argued in previous work that the law's traditional emphasis on biology as key to parentage is harmful to children, driving parents who could provide nurturing adoptive homes away from children in need and keeping children with biological parents who put them at risk of serious abuse and neglect (Bartholet 1999a, 1999b).

The contribution of evolutionary psychology. Sociobiology, or evolutionary psychology, is enjoying something of a revival today, providing new energy for claims that genetics should play a yet more important role in defining parentage than it traditionally has (Wright 1994). Some of its adherents claim that, because of "biological favoritism," child rearing by nonrelatives is "inherently problematic." They say that human beings, like the rest of the animal kingdom, are genetically programmed to produce and to favor their own progeny over others': "It is not that unrelated individuals are unable to do the job of parenting, it is just that they are not as likely to do the job well" (Popenoe 1994, 19). Richard Dawkins, who has done much to popularize evolutionary psychology, describes adoption as a "mistake," a "misfiring of a built-in rule." He claims that "the generous female is doing her own genes no good by caring for the orphan. She is wasting time and energy which she could be investing in the lives of her own kin, particularly future children of her own" (Dawkins 1989, 101). Martin Daly and Margo Wilson, leading proponents of evolutionary psychology, write in their well-known book *Homicide:* "Perhaps the most obvious prediction from a Darwinian view of parental motives is this: Substitute parents will generally tend to care less profoundly for children than natural parents, with the result that children reared by people other than their natural parents will be more often exploited and otherwise at risk. Parental investment is a precious resource, and selection must favor those parental psyches that do not squander it on nonrelatives" (Daly and Wilson 1988, 83). Sexual strategies theory promotes a related claim—that men are genetically programmed to choose women who will faithfully raise their progeny. Thus, when DNA evidence shows that a child a man thought was his biological child is not his, revealing that the woman has betrayed him, he reacts with anger toward both the woman and the child (Buss and Schmitt 1993, 216–18).

Evolutionary theorizing of this kind has been subject to powerful critiques in recent years (Orr 2003; Fodor 2000; Gould and Lewontin 1994). While it does seem likely that biology *matters* in parenting, as the sociobiologists quoted above claim, the important issues are how much it matters, how much factors other than biology—including socialization—matter, and what values we want to promote. Evolutionary theory provides little help in addressing these issues.

Sociobiologists who promote the biological favoritism theory have produced little empirical support for its validity in the realm of human parenting (Orr 2003; Carbone and Cahn 2003). Those claiming the existence of empirical support all point to Daly and Wilson's well-known study of stepparenting (e.g., Pinker 2002). Their study purports to provide empirical grounding for the biological favoritism claim, by demonstrating higher rates of abuse, both physical and sexual, in stepparent households and by stepparents than in households with genetically related parents (Daly and Wilson 1999). However, some highly respected research challenges the generally accepted conclusion that stepparents are disproportionately responsible for abuse (Gelles and Harrop 1991). Even assuming the higher abuse rates claimed, Daly and Wilson's arguments are notably unpersuasive because they fail entirely to address the many obvious factors other than genetics that could explain disproportionate abuse in stepparent households.

A 1997 law review article applying evolutionary theory to child abuse also relies on Daly and Wilson's stepparent data as proof, but acknowledges the potential validity of alternative explanatory theories. Author Owen Jones claims that policy makers ignore evolutionary theory in devising policy and argues that appropriate deference to evolutionary theory would result in policies premised on the assumption that adults will prefer genetically related children (Jones 1997, 1117, 1200–1204, 1221–22). Although Jones makes only the relatively modest claim that genetics should count for *more* in policy making related to parenting, even this claim is unpersuasive. He fails to acknowledge the degree to which current policy is already heavily influenced by the assumption that genetics matters, even if this is more because of what policy makers understand as "natural" than because they have mastered and are believers in evolutionary theory. There is, after all, a rather common assumption that "blood is thicker than water," which has translated into laws and policies placing significant emphasis on genetics in all issues related to parentage. Jones makes no persuasive showing that genetics should count for more than it already does.

The stepparent evidence is, in any event, countered by powerful evidence that looks in the opposite direction, which these sociobiologists fail to address in any significant way. Adoption studies show adoptive parent-child relationships working essentially as well as biological parent-child relationships. Daly and Wilson (1988, 1999) admit that adoption apparently does work well, without ever adequately explaining how this could be true if genetics is so central to parenting capacity. Jones (1997, 1207) similarly makes only the most modest attempt to explain away adoption's success.

Carbone and Cahn's analysis of studies of fathers who move from one adult relationship to another show that these men seem to care more for the non-related children with whom they are living than the related children they have left behind. Apparently, any "biological favoritism" that may exist is outweighed by the adult relationship factor (Carbone and Cahn 2003). These authors show that biological favoritism theorists typically fail to take into account the complexity of human beings and their institutional lives: "Humans act not just through direct provisions for their children and indifference (or even hostility) toward others but through the creation of complex customs and institutions that instill values and habits including altruism and selfishness. The trick in using sociobiology to make sense of parental behavior therefore lies in identifying the competing tendencies and the possible trade-offs among them" (1028–29). They show the complexity of trying to figure out, based on sociobiology's insights, available empirical evidence, and efforts to predict the effect of societal norms on human behavior, what parentage-defining policies would maximize the likelihood of providing children with nurturing parents.

Biology may matter. Human beings may be genetically programmed to prefer their genetic offspring over other children. But factors other than biology also matter in shaping parenting desires and capacities. Social conditioning has a huge impact. Moreover, it seems likely that we would maximize human happiness if we were to shape our culture in ways that reduced rather than reinforced any natural tendency to prefer our genetic relatives over others.

Increasingly, even sociobiologists who promote the biological favoritism thesis admit or even assert that the *is* is not the same as the *ought,* that culture matters, that humans are different from other animals, and that part of the point of human existence is to overcome nature (Wright 1994; Wilson 1975; Ridley 2003). Dawkins writes that human beings have the capacity to defy their genetic programming and to cultivate altruism deliberately (Dawkins 1989, 200–201). Robert Wright argues that an important point of understanding our genetic nature is to figure out how to move beyond it toward conscience, sympathy, and love for unrelated others (Wright 1994, 77–79).

Biology in its place. Thus, for many reasons, I think we should reject the various voices proclaiming that DNA is and should be the key to determining true parentage. However, I am not yet ready to jettison biology entirely as a factor in defining parentage. I worry about the way in which our society seems to be doing just this in the realm of reproductive technology. I think it will be better, in general, for parents and children if we encourage adults to conceive children with the intention of raising rather than selling or otherwise disposing of them, and if children are raised by biologically linked parents rather than biological strangers. There are many reasons to think that this kind of parenting regime will be better for children, some of which I have explored elsewhere (Bartholet 1999a, 223–29).

Commercialization of reproduction and of parenting rights creates risks of exploitation and of devaluing both parenting relationships and children. Apart from commercialization, treating the creation of a new life as a relative nonevent for the creator—an act that does not necessarily entail any long-term responsibility for the life created—seems unlikely to encourage, in society generally, the kind of committed nurturing that children need. Adoption works extremely well for those who choose to pursue it and for their adopted children, but it still seems reasonable to think that most adults might do better parenting genetically related children than unrelated children. Many are likely to find it easier to relate to children somewhat like themselves, and genetic links increase the chance for similarities. Also, a weak version of the biological favoritism thesis seems plausible and fits with a broadly shared sense that it is "natural" to want to create and raise genetic progeny. It should be possible to cater to this desire while simultaneously encouraging love for unrelated others. Finally, using biology as one guiding factor helps keep the state out of decision making in this important area, thus contributing to the values of autonomy and diversity that U.S. society deems so important. So in my view we should count biology as one factor among others in defining parentage.

Children also have at least some significant interest in knowing their biological heritage, certainly in a society such as ours that places a high value on
that heritage. (But also, if there is something natural about wanting to create
and raise genetic progeny, there may be something natural about wanting to
connect to one's genetic forebears [Bartholet 1999a, 227–29]). And, if it is important to encourage adults to act responsibly when they create life, we should
encourage them to demonstrate care and concern even for those children
who have been assigned to others for primary parenting purposes. So in cases
where it does not make sense for the genetic parent to be the legal parent, we
should consider giving children at least an informational link with the genetic
parent. This is complicated, because in a society that overvalues genetics, as
I believe ours does, creating that informational link risks exacerbating this
problem, adding to the sense that genetics is overwhelmingly important. It
may also create pressure to define the biological parent as the legal parent.
However, we need to move forward to a stage where we can put biology in its
place and keep it there. We need to recognize that, in some situations, the genetic contributor is a relevant person but a nonparent, and the social parent
is a fully real legal parent.

Best Interests of the Child: A Central Factor

Children's best interests *should* be, as we generally say they are, the guiding
principle for the law in all matters involving children. This is not because adult
interests do not matter but because children are not able to fight for their interests, either in the absence of law or in designing law, so there is always a
major risk that their interests will not be protected. The interests of the larger
society are also served by treating its children well, because they are the future
(Bartholet 1999b, 60).

Our legal system's claim that the best interests of children serve as the guiding principle for all law relating to children is often ignored in reality. Thoughtful observers of the law's effects regularly remark on this problem. In my own
work, I have seen it demonstrated in our restrictive regulation of adoption,
which drives prospective parents away from the children who need homes; in
our free-market approach to reproductive technologies, which exposes children to health and other risks (Bartholet 1999a); and in our emphasis on family preservation in the face of child abuse and neglect, which protects parents
at the expense of their children (Bartholet 1999b). Several national commis-
sions have examined our treatment of children and found it wanting, one des-

ignating child abuse and neglect a "national emergency" (U.S. Advisory Board 1990). The problem is not uniquely American; civilizations throughout history have subjected children to various forms of horrible abuse (ten Bensel, Rheinberger, and Radbill 1997).

Because children cannot participate in reshaping the law or in actively protecting their own interests, and because their interests have been inadequately protected by the law throughout history, we need to make a self-conscious effort to take their best interests seriously in all law reform efforts. We must be suspicious of the claim that protecting adult parenting rights equates with protecting children, a claim that constitutes a major rationale for the deference our system has traditionally paid to parental rights.

This means that in defining parentage, obviously a central issue for children's well-being, we need to make some basic changes in the way the law allocates rights. Typically the law packages parental rights with parental responsibilities but in the end gives undue emphasis to rights. The law talks of children's best interests as determinative but in the end generally lets adults' interests trump children's. We must adjust the law to place greater emphasis on *parental responsibilities* and *children's rights to receive responsible parenting.*

Related Rules of the Road

With the above as the core principles, we can move on to some modestly more specific guidelines for an appropriate parent-picking system.

Provide children early in life with permanent parents. Developmental psychology, social science, and common sense all demonstrate clearly that children need nurturing parents from early infancy onward and that they need permanency (e.g., Goldstein et al. 1996). This reality about children's needs has a different quality than the reality some sociobiologists claim about adults' preferences to parent biologically related children. First, there is a great deal of empirical evidence showing that children do better with permanent parenting and, as discussed above, little or none showing that biologically related parents do better than unrelated parents. Second, there is no reason to think that we would create a better society by trying to condition children to live without permanent nurturing, whereas, as discussed above, there is reason to think that we would do well to try to temper any tendency to prefer relatives over others. Finally, we are unlikely to succeed in changing human nature to the point of enabling children to surmount their need for stability in nurturing relationships. Many children are able to survive and even thrive despite disruption in familial relationships, but it does not seem plausible that we could create a world in which most children would do as well under such conditions as they would with permanent nurturing parents. By contrast, we should be able to condition adults not to create dependent children unless they are willing to stay the course, and adoption studies demonstrate that adults are capable of parenting unrelated children very successfully, with relation to both their own and their children's needs (Bartholet 1999a).

Ideally our legal system should decide definitively who will be a child's parents from birth through entry into adulthood (Carbone and Cahn 2003). The new Uniform Parentage Act (2000, §§ 607, 609) would improve current law by providing children with earlier resolution of parentage, but it does not go far enough in this respect. It allows proceedings to be brought for resolving disputed parentage in a variety of situations for up to two years after a child's birth and allows "presumed fathers" in certain situations to bring proceedings at any time.

An appropriate parentage system could look to any of a variety of factors, including many that the current system considers: who the birth parent is, who the genetic parents are, who the intended parents are, whether the child is born in a marriage, whether there is any established parenting relationship, and what parenting relationship has the best prospects for being ongoing, permanent, and nurturing. More important than the weight given to particular substantive factors is that the system have clear rules establishing permanent parenthood early in the child's life. So, for example, the system could mandate that if a child is born in a marriage, the husband will be the permanent father. Or it could declare that all children must be genetically tested at birth and matched if possible with their genetic fathers, who will then be declared their legal permanent fathers even if the mother is married to another. Or it could say that, although such testing should be done, it would be designed simply to give children information about their genetic heritage, leaving their birth mother's husband as their legal permanent father. Or the law could provide for some variation on the above themes.

Policy makers should choose among such systems with a view toward maximizing the chances of giving children, at or close to birth, a father who will be a permanent nurturing parent, and they should design the rules so that parenthood, once established, cannot be easily dissolved. The model for any limited escape route should be surrender for adoption, whereby, if it clearly makes sense for a new parent to take over for an inadequate one, the original parent is allowed to surrender parenting rights and the new parent is allowed to adopt and become the full legal parent. Completely unacceptable is the unfortunately frequent modern phenomenon of allowing men with established parenting relationships to exit those relationships solely because they have proof that they are not the biological fathers. They may not be *worthy* fathers, but they should be held responsible as legal fathers. Although these fathers' unfortunate children may get little more than support payments, future children will benefit from parentage rules designed to condition men to understand that once they take on parenting responsibilities they cannot easily shed them.

Provide children with nurturing parents. This idea sounds obvious, but the point is that in choosing between different parental candidates, we should put a very high value on finding a parent who will establish a powerful emotional, caretaking relationship. For example, in choosing between the genetic father and the husband of the birth mother, we should design our legal system to maximize the chances of selecting a father who is likely to provide *ongoing* high-quality nurturing (Carbone and Cahn 2003).

We should also be prepared to surrender the traditional idea that parents provide all the financial support that children need. At present, parentage policy is unduly driven by the felt need to find a bill payer. Genetic tests are used to pursue deadbeat dads with the goal of getting financial support. We should not choose "the father" based primarily on the need to find a source of financial support. Obviously it is problematic from the child's perspective to be given a father who has no interest in the nurturing aspect of parenting, simply because the man might have wages available to be garnished. If another man is available who seems suitable for the nurturing aspect of parenting, we should consider him for the parental role regardless of whether he can take care of financial support responsibilities. We could look to the state to take on more support responsibilities in cases where a child's nurturing parents cannot provide for the child's financial needs. Alternatively, we could pursue genetic fathers incapable of nurturing for financial support without giving them parenting rights. Adults should not be seen as having a necessary right to have the entire parenting package or none of it. Parents' and children's rights should not be seen as necessarily reciprocal, with fathers who provide financial support entitled as a matter of absolute right to receive the benefits of the parenting relationship because the child who receives support is deemed to owe the father something. We should place a higher value on children's rights to a nurturing upbringing than on parents' rights to control their progeny.

Hold parents responsible. Adults are in the position of making decisions to create children and thus to create children's dependency—decisions in which the children at issue can play no part. Accordingly, it is appropriate to hold adults responsible for children (Carbone and Cahn 2003).

We should feel free to hold men responsible regardless of whether they were in some way misled into parenthood by women. Children should not be penalized in a way that denies them fundamental nurturing and support because of the actions of their mothers. We already apply this principle in the area of biological parenting. We hold men responsible for children they conceive even if they were deceived by the mothers' false claims that they were using birth control. We hold men responsible for children they conceive even if they had wanted the woman to have an abortion but she refused. We hold men responsible for the lives they participate in creating, and this is right.

However, some men have twisted this principle of responsibility to avoid responsibility. Male resentment at being required to provide financial support for the children they have produced is a major factor in the new move to dissolve parenting responsibility in situations where men have genetic proof that they did not produce the children at issue. Men claim that if a DNA match alone can be used to force them into parenthood, then the absence of a DNA match should enable them to escape parenthood.

Such arguments ignore the different ways in which men (and women) can create children for whose dependency they are morally responsible. The high court in Massachusetts made this principle quite clear in the *In re Paternity of Cheryl* (2001) case discussed above. A few months after Cheryl's birth, the man named by her mother as the father formally acknowledged paternity. He then functioned as a noncustodial visitation and support father for several years. He apparently thought that he was the genetic father for some of that time, although later he suspected that he might not be. Five and a half years after the paternity judgment, just after the court ordered an increase in his support obligation, he moved for genetic testing and for revision of the paternity judgment should the testing indicate he was not the genetic father. Although this motion was denied, he took Cheryl for testing on his own, and when the results revealed she was not his genetic child, he again moved the court to relieve him of any parental support obligations, now some six years after the paternity judgment. The Massachusetts high court held him to his parental responsibilities. Given that the situation was parallel to the biological parentage cases discussed above, only an undue obsession with biology as the basis for parentage could explain the outrage hurled at the court by enraged men and other critics. The child in this case grew up as this man's child, calling him "daddy" and receiving not just his financial support but his parental visits. The man created this child as his child and is responsible for her dependency on him, much as the man who contributes sperm to create a child is responsible for that child's existence and related dependency. He should be held responsible under law. It is irrelevant, as the Massachusetts court found, whether the mother tricked him into thinking the child was biologically his or not. He could have avoided creating the dependency, in this case by getting genetic tests done at birth, if biology were so important to him, and then deciding not to act like a parent when those tests showed him not to be the genetic father. By contrast, the child had no choice in whether or not to become his child.

We should also feel free to hold parents responsible without believing that we have to give them reciprocal rights in all cases. As discussed above, in some situations it would be appropriate to hold men responsible for financial support without giving them parenting rights. We might also want to hold genetic parents responsible for providing biological heritage information to children who are being raised by other parents, without giving the genetic parents any reciprocal rights. We might decide, as some countries have, to give not just adopted children but also the children of reproductive technology the right to access identifying as well as nonidentifying information about their genetic parents. This does not mean that we have to create rights for the genetic contributors to get a piece of the parenting pie, by giving them, for example, visitation rights during the child's growing-up period. Again, adults and the children they create are not in a state of equality appropriate for reciprocity. Adults who agree to a deal whereby one sells his sperm so that another can obtain a child make their deal with one another, without consulting the child-to-be. If children born by virtue of this kind of arrangement have a significant interest in accessing information about their birth heritage, then we should provide it, based on the principle that adults are to be held responsible to the children they create.

In the same way, if we make a birth mother's husband the legal father of a child born during the marriage, we might choose to give the child a right to access birth heritage information by requiring genetic testing at birth and recording the information. We should not feel compelled to give a genetic father so identified any visitation rights simply because he is held responsible to his progeny to the degree of having his identity revealed.

Give family privacy its due; or, don't unduly knock the nuclear family. It is popular in many quarters to argue that our societal obsession with the nuclear family is responsible for a range of family problems, and that if one or two parents are good for children, three or four would be even better. Here, more may be less, or at least less good. Family privacy in the parenting context means, among other things, that parents are left alone by the state to raise their children, with the state intervening only to insist on certain minimal protections such as vaccination and education and, beyond that, intervening only when parents are proven unfit. This aspect of family privacy is justified in part by the understanding that children will generally be better off if their parents have primary decision-making responsibility and in part by the values our society places on autonomy and diversity (Goldstein et al. 1996; Davis 1994, 1370–71).

Family privacy gets sacrificed to an enormous degree with divorce. When parents split up, both are treated by law as ongoing parents. One may be the primary and one the visitation parent, but both have parenting rights, enforceable by courts. Increasingly, the law permits and even mandates joint parenting after divorce, with parents given equal decision-making power and often equal parenting time, posing the likelihood of an ongoing need for courts to resolve disputes. When courts are called on to decide which of two warring parents should prevail, they are forced into the intimacy of the family and required to decide how the child should be raised, in direct conflict with family privacy principles. Courts will necessarily be second-guessing one parent based on the other parent's demands. The child will not experience the kind of stable parental authority that many think central to children's best interests. It is for these reasons that the authors of the famous *Beyond the Best Interests of the Child* (Goldstein, Freud, and Solnit 1973, 90–92; Goldstein et al. 1996) argued that sole custody should be given to one parent after divorce, so that one parent could have exclusive authority and postdivorce families would not surrender classic family autonomy.

Modern life presents us with many situations in which children might be deemed to have a multiplicity of parents—one set of social parents and one, or two, or three biological parents. A child born in the context of marriage can have a husband father as well as a sperm father, if the child was conceived in the wife's nonmarital relationship or by artificial insemination. A child born by gestational surrogacy can have an egg parent, a sperm parent, a pregnancy parent, and a couple of social/rearing parents.

Today we may know who the genetic parents of a child are, because those parents can so easily get genetic tests done. Law may in any event insist that we know, on the grounds that genetic heritage information is important for children. We need to decide whether we want to make all these arguable parents legal parents in any sense—whether we want to give all of them part of the parenting rights pie. We could give all noncustodial "parents" legal visitation rights, if they choose to ask for and exercise them. But we do not have to, and I think we should not. There is real wisdom behind the family privacy presumption, even if it has been taken too far in many respects, putting children at undue risk of abuse and neglect because the state is so reluctant to intervene in the family. The U.S. Supreme Court recently affirmed the importance of letting a child's parents decide what is in their child's best interests and the related right to decide when and whether to allow visitation by others, rather than permitting the state to impose visitation by concededly loving grandparents in the absence of a powerful reason to interfere with the parents' judgment (*Troxel v. Granville* 2000). Children deserve to grow up, if at all possible, with parents in charge, rather than in the shadow of the court. We put the children of divorce in the latter, less-than-ideal situation, feeling compelled to do so because of their parents' "rights" and the often significant parenting relationships already developed before divorce. There is no such need to put all children with the multiple parents that the modern world may produce in that situation. And, if we are to be guided by the best interests of children, we will not do so.

Conclusion

Modern developments present us with many new and complex issues in defining parentage. It is important to focus on the basics. The key issues are social, political, and legal, not scientific. *We can do what we will.* DNA tests cannot force us to decide that one person is a "real" parent and another is not. *We should do what will serve children.* What children need is ongoing, stable, nurturing relationships with parents, whether or not those parents are genetic relatives.

ACKNOWLEDGMENT

An earlier version of this chapter appeared as E. Bartholet, "Guiding Principles for Picking Parents," *Harvard Women's Law Journal* 27 (2004): 323–44.

BIBLIOGRAPHY

American Law Institute. 2002. *Principles of the Law of Family Dissolution: Analysis and Recommendations,* § 2.03. Newark: The Institute.

Anderlik, M. R., and M. A. Rothstein. 2002. DNA-based identity testing and the future of the family: A research agenda. *American Journal of Law and Medicine* 28:215–32.

Bartholet, E. 1999a. *Family Bonds: Adoption, Infertility, and the New World of Child Production.* Boston: Beacon Press.

———. 1999b. *Nobody's Children: Abuse and Neglect, Foster Drift, and the Adoption Alternative.* Boston: Beacon Press.

Buss, D. M., and D. P. Schmitt. 1993. Sexual strategies theory: An evolutionary perspective on human mating. *Psychology Review* 100:204–32.

Carbone, J., and N. Cahn. 2003. Which ties bind? Redefining the parent-child relationship in an age of genetic certainty. *William and Mary Bill of Rights Journal* 11:1011–70.

Daly, M., and M. Wilson. 1988. *Homicide.* New York: Aldine de Gruyter.

———. 1999. *The Truth about Cinderella: A Darwinian View of Parental Love.* New Haven: Yale University Press.

Davis, P. C. 1994. Contested images of family values: The role of the state. *Harvard Law Review* 107:1348–73.

Dawkins, R. 1989. *The Selfish Gene,* 2nd ed. New York: Oxford University Press.

Doran v. Doran. 2003. 820 A.2d 1279, 1281 (Pa. Super. Ct.).

Fodor, J. 2000. *The Mind Doesn't Work That Way: The Scope and Limits of Computational Psychology.* Cambridge: MIT Press.

Gelles, R. J., and J. W. Harrop. 1991. The risk of abusive violence among children with nongenetic caretakers. *FamilyRelations* 40:78–83.

Goldstein, J., A. Freud, and A. J. Solnit. 1973. *Beyond the Best Interests of the Child.* New York: Free Press.

Goldstein, J., A. J. Solnit, S. Goldstein, and A. Freud. 1996. *The Best Interests of the Child: The Least Detrimental Alternative.* New York: Free Press.

Gould, S. J., and R. C. Lewontin. 1994. The Spandrels of San Marco and the Panglossian paradigm: A critique of the adaptationist programme. In *Conceptual Issues in Evolutionary Biology,* 2nd ed., ed. E. Sober, 73–70. Cambridge: MIT Press, Bradford Books.

Harvard Law Review. 2003. Changing realities of parenthood: The law's response to the evolving American family and emerging reproductive technologies. Developments in the Law: IV. 116:2052–74.

In re Paternity of Cheryl. 2001. 746 N.E.2d 488, 492 (Mass.).

Jones, O. D. 1997. Evolutionary analysis in law: An introduction and application to child abuse. *North Carolina Law Review* 75:1117–1242.

Michael H. v. Gerald D. 1989. 491 U.S. 110 (1989), *reh'g denied,* 492 U.S. 937.

Orr, H. A. 2003. *Darwinian Storytelling.* New York: New York Review Books.

Pinker, S. 2002. *The Blank Slate: The Modern Denial of Human Nature.* New York: Penguin Putnam.

Popenoe, D. 1994. The evolution of marriage and the problem of stepfamilies. In *Stepfamilies: Who Benefits? Who Does Not?* ed. A. Booth and J. Dunn, 3–27. Hillsdale, NJ: Erlbaum.

Ridley, M. 2003. What makes you who you are: Which is stronger—nature or nurture? *Time* 161 (2 June): 54–62.

Roberts, P. 2004. Truth and consequences: Part I: Disestablishing the paternity of non-marital children. Center for Law and Social Policy. www.clasp.org/DMS/Documents/ 1046817229.69/truth_and_consequences1.pdf (accessed 15 February 2004).

ten Bensel, R. W., M. Rheinberger, and S. Radbill. 1997. Children in a world of violence: The roots of child maltreatment. In *The Battered Child,* 5th ed., ed. M. E. Helfer, R. Kempe, and D. Krugman, 3–28. Chicago: University of Chicago Press.

Troxel v. Granville. 2000. 530 U.S. 57.

U.S. Advisory Board on Child Abuse and Neglect, U.S. Department of Health and Human Services. 1990. *Child Abuse and Neglect: Critical First Steps in Response to a National Emergency.* Washington, DC: The Board.

Welstead, M. 2003. The influence of human rights and cultural issues. In *International Survey of Family Law,* ed. A. Bainham, 143–62. Bristol: Family Law.

Wilson, E. O. 1975. Human decency is animal. *New York Times,* 12 October.

Wright, R. 1994. *The Moral Animal: Evolutionary Psychology and Everyday Life.* New York: Pantheon Books.

CHAPTER NINE

Reforming American Paternity Procedures

Jeffrey A. Parness, J.D.

The exploration of genetic ties and legal parenthood in this chapter focuses on parentage at the time of live birth in the United States of a child conceived the old-fashioned way, through consensual sexual intercourse. So, *biological, natural,* or *genetic* mother herein refers to a woman who is both a genetically tied and a gestational mother. For parents, legal designations usually result in parental rights, including parental opportunity interests (usually relevant only for men, typically unwed natural fathers) and child-rearing rights. They also result in parental responsibilities (including child support). Assignment of responsibilities need not also prompt significant rights. For children, designations of legal parenthood spur other rights (e.g., inheritance) but few or no responsibilities.

In exploring genetic ties and legal parenthood, I examine differences between parental rights and responsibilities and between legal maternity and paternity. The major thesis is that old-fashioned pregnancies require new-fashioned paternity laws. Reforms are both necessitated and facilitated by recent scientific advances. Existing laws too often unfairly eliminate parental rights or assign parental responsibilities to unwed natural fathers. The chief concern here is with procedure, not substance. In this chapter, I support the proposition that legal paternity "should be determined . . . consistent with orderly procedure without unnecessary involvement in procedural quirks, complications and limitations" (*Gunn v. Cavanaugh* 1965).

Unfortunately, procedural quirks often arise because of the troublesome governmental treatment of maternal conduct, frequently prompting cries about duped dads. Sympathy, however, is often not forthcoming, perhaps because of a confusion with deadbeat dads. Yet "screwed" dads should be distinguished from dads who "screw up." Some natural fathers do merit our sympathy, including perhaps the lonely boy described in the following song recorded by Heart, entitled *All I Want to Do Is Make Love to You:*

It was a rainy night
When he came into sight,

. . . .

So I pulled up alongside
And I offered him a ride.

. . . .

I didn't ask him his name,
This lonely boy in the rain.
Fate tell me it's right,
Is this love at first sight?

. . . .

All I wanna do is make love to you
Say you will
You want me too

. . . .

So we found this hotel,
It was a place I knew well
We made magic that night.
Oh, he did everything right
He brought the woman out of me,
So many times, easily
And in the morning when he woke all
I left him was a note
I told him
I am the flower you are the seed
We walked in the garden
We planted a tree
Don't try to find me,
Please don't you dare
Just live in my memory,
You'll always be there

. . . .

Oh, oooh, we made love
Love like strangers
. . . .

Then it happened one day,
We came round the same way
You can imagine his surprise
When he saw his own eyes
I said please, please understand
I'm in love with another man
And what he couldn't give me
Was the one little thing that you can

All I wanna do is make love to you
. . . .

How should parentage laws treat the child, the mother, and the two men in this story: the Lonely Boy, and the Other Man? Should any adult male interests ever be wholly dependent on maternal conduct? How should laws treat the acts of the woman before and after the birth? Should it matter whether the Lonely Boy or the Other Man was duped? Should legal procedures depend on the age or economic status of the Other Man, the Lonely Boy, or the woman; the fact or timing of a marriage of the woman to the Other Man; or the places where conception, pregnancy, birth, or child rearing occurred? In reviewing the American legal landscape, I will focus particularly on the parental opportunity interests, child-rearing rights, and child-support responsibilities of the Lonely Boy and the Other Man.

Overview of American State Parentage Laws

Unquestionably, public policy throughout the United States supports early, complete, accurate, informed, and conclusive designations of legal parenthood at the time of birth. For most women and for many men, such designations are founded on genetic ties. A 1992 federal study, *Supporting Our Children*, said this about the importance of early designation: "Parentage determination does more than provide genealogical clues to a child's background; it establishes fundamental emotional, social, legal and economic ties between parent and child. It is a prerequisite to securing financial support for the child and to developing the heightened emotional support the child derives from enforceable custody and visitation rights. Parentage determination also unlocks the door to government provided dependent's benefits, inheritance, and an accurate medical history for the child." (U.S. Commission on Interstate Child Support 1992, 120).

Although all parentage designations at birth are important, legal standards guiding maternity and paternity differ in both substance and procedure. Thus, for federal constitutional parental rights, the U.S. Supreme Court has recognized differences between natural mothers and natural fathers of children conceived through consensual sexual intercourse. In a dissent in 1979, which has since been widely used, Justice Potter Stewart wrote,

> Parental rights do not spring full-blown from the biological connection between parent and child. They require relationships more enduring. The mother carries and bears the child, and in this sense her parental relationship is clear. The validity of the father's parental claims must be gauged by other measures. By tradition, the primary measure has been the legitimate familial relationship he creates with the child by marriage with the mother . . . In some circumstances the actual relationship between father and child may suffice to create in the . . . father parental interests (*Caban v. Mohammed* 1979).

The differing treatment of natural mothers and fathers extends beyond the required forms of "enduring" relationships. In 2001, when exploring the different procedures for women and men seeking parental rights by proving genetic ties, Justice Anthony Kennedy explained it thus:

> The first governmental interest to be served is the importance of assuring that a biological parent-child relationship exists. In the case of the mother, the relation is verifiable from the birth itself. The mother's status is documented in most instances by the birth certificate or hospital records and the witnesses who attest to her having given birth.
>
> In the case of the father, the uncontestable fact is that he need not be present at the birth. If he is present, furthermore, that circumstance is not incontrovertible proof of fatherhood . . . Fathers and mothers are not similarly situated with regard to the proof of biological parenthood. The imposition of a different set of rules for making that legal determination with respect to fathers and mothers is neither surprising nor troublesome from a constitutional perspective (*Nguyen v. INS* 2001).

Both Justice Stewart and Justice Kennedy each recognize the significant legal differences between natural mothers and fathers in many settings. Justice Stewart declares that parental rights require more than "biological connection," but he finds that the necessary "enduring" relationship for a mother arises from biology alone, in that she "carries and bears the child." For a man, he says, often there must be an "actual relationship between father and child." Justice Stewart also hints that such an actual relationship, developed as soon as humanly possible, may still be insufficient for certain natural fathers. For example, it may be insufficient if a natural mother is married to another man at the time of conception, pregnancy, or birth and that man wishes to parent within an intact family (*Michael H. v. Gerald D.* 1989). Thus all natural mothers, but not all natural fathers, have "enduring" relationships with their children that prompt parental rights.

At times, for a natural father, no actual parent-child relationship or genetic tie is necessary to establish an "enduring" relationship. Justice Stewart himself noted that an "enduring" male connection may be proven in some states solely by marriage to the natural mother at the time of the child's birth. Elsewhere, presumptions without marriage at the time of birth can spur "enduring" relationships, as with men who were married to mothers at the time of conception or for some time during the pregnancy. In some states an alleged natural father can also establish an "enduring" relationship under law simply through one or more of the following: (1) listing his name on a state-established paternity register; (2) being named on the birth certificate; (3) swearing to paternity under oath or otherwise acknowledging paternity; (4) procuring a court order adjudicating paternity; and (5) providing child support.

Whether or not substantive legal paternity norms require proof of actual relationships or genetic ties, many would-be fathers will require the aid of natural mothers to establish legal paternity. Moms can flee, fail to disclose a pregnancy, abandon a newborn, or misrepresent their sexual encounters. And in at least some settings in which genetic ties matter, natural mothers may deny natural fathers access to needed scientific testing, thereby effectively denying the men their "unique opportunity" to "grasp" parenthood (*Lehr v. Robertson* 1983). Such testing denials are often respected under law regardless of a mother's motives. Further, some paternity laws allow others, such as the husbands of natural mothers, to block alleged natural fathers from testing and thus from establishing "enduring" parent-child relationships. By contrast, it is unimaginable that any person, including a natural father, could ever deny a natural mother her "unique opportunity" to rear her child.

For legal paternity, although not for legal maternity, context is often crucial. In a single state, maternity and paternity at the time of birth are important in many situations, such as for child support duties, child custody and visitation rights, criminal law duties, and remedial rights under tort or probate laws. There often are different approaches to legal paternity, but not to legal maternity. Thus the substantive standards for legal paternity can vary for civil child support and for criminal child support. Only under the criminal laws does the alleged legal father need to know before a lawsuit of his child's existence and of his responsibility to support the child under law. Also, the procedures employed for designating legal paternity may vary. In the child custody setting, only the potential legal father, the natural mother, the child, and the state (especially if it is providing child support) may have standing to litigate legal paternity; in the inheritance setting, more actual and alleged family members may also have standing. American paternity laws also vary widely from state to state, even in a single setting. For example, there are differing substantive law standards in the child custody setting for rebuttals of paternity presumptions grounded on marriage (Glennon 2000; Kaplan 2000). There are also differing procedural law standards for birth certificate designations of paternity that guide parental rights in such settings as adoption and visitation.

Finally, legal paternity can be designated to assign parental responsibilities to a man who is not then entitled (and may never be, or may never have been, entitled) to parental rights. Thus, under laws based solely on genetic ties, a man who fails to establish a parent-child relationship prompting child-rearing rights may be pursued for child support long after the birth. These proceedings can even involve a man who had earlier been denied access to genetic testing in his attempt to secure parental rights. An award and the payment of child support later in life may, but need not, revive any real chance for child rearing. Of course, for natural mothers parental rights and responsibilities as of the time of birth are clearly recognized at the birth.

Heartless Paternity Procedures

Given these premises, how would existing state laws treat the parental opportunity interests and child-rearing rights of the people in the song: the mother, the Other Man, and the Lonely Boy? Are any of the procedures unfair to the mother, the Lonely Boy, the Other Man, or the child?

The mother would always be accorded the "opportunity" to rear her child. While she might fail to take advantage of that opportunity, any postbirth failure would typically involve her own intentional, or at least very culpable, acts (e.g., abandonment), which would not include deceit about the circumstances of her pregnancy (directed at the natural father, any husband or boyfriend, any other male, or the state). Any prebirth maternal acts prompting loss of child-rearing rights at the time of birth usually would also encompass highly culpable acts, such as significant drug or alcohol use during pregnancy or significant and proven abuse of another child that will likely be replicated. As with postbirth acts, relevant prebirth acts usually do not encompass deceit about male genetic ties or about the pregnancy itself.

The Other Man usually would be accorded presumptive legal paternity status and thus parental rights, as long as he was married to the mother at birth. Marriage at some point during the pregnancy, but not at birth, might also suffice. When he first knew (or should have known) of the circumstance of the pregnancy or birth, or if he ever knew, is typically irrelevant. The presumption may be rebuttable. Where rebuttable, the circumstances are defined by statute or compelled by state constitutional law; they often, but not always, disfavor the natural father—the Lonely Boy. To date, there is no major federal constitutional law precedent compelling even an opportunity for rebuttal by the natural father. If the presumption is rebutted by the natural father, the Other Man can lose parental rights even though he fully grasped the opportunity for child rearing, desires that his parenthood continue, and is a fit parent. Child-rearing rights may be lost by the Other Man even when his continuing parenthood is in the child's best interests. At times the marital presumption can also be rebutted by other than natural fathers. The woman, the Other Man, or the government (seeking reimbursement for child support it has paid) may be entitled to overcome the presumption long after birth (as when the woman and the Other Man divorce), even if rebuttal was unavailable to the natural father and even if the natural father (now possibly subject to child support obligations) had not known earlier of his genetic ties.

If the Other Man in the song was not married to the mother before or at the time of birth, his parental rights are more fragile. Legal paternity may be unavailable, or subject to loss, even if he always believed, quite reasonably, that the child was genetically tied to him and he successfully stepped up to parenthood through filling out governmental forms or through effective child rearing. Thus, under some state laws, after a breakup of unwed couples, the mother can disestablish the legal paternity of the man simply through genetic testing, even when the man's name appeared on the birth certificate and even though the man actually parented the child for some time. Such disestablishment can follow a mother's romantic relationship with a Lonely Boy or with some other man (especially if he wishes to adopt). Under other state laws the mother is estopped.

The Lonely Boy in the song has little real opportunity to establish legal paternity and to grasp parenthood. Notwithstanding her note left after the night of "magic" when the boy did "everything right," the mother had no legal duty to inform him of her possible or actual pregnancy or of any later birth. One state statute says, "An unmarried biological father, by virtue of the fact that he has engaged in a sexual relationship with a woman, is deemed to be on notice that a pregnancy and an adoption proceeding . . . may occur, and has a duty to protect his own rights and interests" (Idaho Code § 16-1505(2)). Further, even had the Lonely Boy come "round the same way" during the pregnancy and then been deceived by the natural mother, his chances for establishing legal paternity immediately after a later, postbirth encounter with the mother and child would be remote, at best, although he only then learned of the likely genetic ties. Frequently, too much time has passed and any attempt to seize the parental opportunity interest is deemed too late. Yet should the mother, or the child, or the state determine later (even after such encounters and deceit) to hold the Lonely Boy financially responsible for child support, their causes would be well-received in most courts.

Such treatment of natural fathers is unfair. Reforms are necessary, particularly for an unwed natural father who is denied any real opportunity shortly after birth to establish an "enduring" parent-child relationship with a child born to an unwed natural mother. Reforms are especially important when such a relationship would also likely serve the child's best interests and when the same man can be pursued much later for child support.

Paternity Procedure Reforms

Without changing substantive law guidelines, American legal paternity procedures can most easily be improved through reforms of birth certificate laws. If birth certificates completed at the time of birth, or shortly thereafter, more fully spoke to legal paternity interests, including the interests of husbands, natural fathers, actual fathers, and adopting fathers, societal and individual needs for early, complete, and formidable, if not conclusive, legal paternity designations would be better promoted. Inquiries into legal paternity long after birth could more frequently use earlier certificates, thereby avoiding duplication, excessive expense, and the undermining of settled expectations. How might birth certificate procedures be reformed? The following suggestions initially speak to possible state law changes, as neither federal laws nor local laws historically have regulated birth certificate procedures or such related matters as paternity acknowledgments and paternity adjudications. State parentage law reforms in other areas have been greatly facilitated through the use of uniform standards proposed by such groups as the National Conference of Commissioners on Uniform State Laws (e.g., the Uniform Parentage Act), but no adequate model birth certificate provisions as yet exist.

In the United States, a birth certificate usually is completed under state law shortly after birth. It normally contains either the names or the signatures of the woman and man designated as the child's parents. Nearly always, the woman named is the natural mother of a child born as a result of consensual sexual intercourse. For fathers, birth certificates differ. Often they simply reflect the marriage of the woman to a man, with no explicit reference to genetic ties, though there may be an applicable presumption. For an unwed mother, the designation of male parentage based on genetic ties often is not verified, as when based solely on the written and unsworn statements of the alleged mother and father. When affidavits are required, more typically when mothers are unmarried, little is generally done to ensure their accuracy. In circumstances where birth certificates designate male parentage based only on legal presumptions involving marriage, and where the presumptions could be rebutted by unwed natural fathers, there are typically no governmental or private efforts to encourage the identification and notification of unwed fathers or to inform the mothers of possible male parental opportunity interests, even when there is evidence of no genetic ties between husband and child.

Birth certificates can also be incomplete, as when information on male parentage is missing. Seemingly, the father most frequently remains unnamed if the mother is unwed at the time of birth. The numbers of incomplete birth certificates have increased in the past forty years as the numbers of births to unwed mothers have risen sharply. In 1960, in the United States, about 5 percent of children were born to unwed mothers; by 1994, about a third of all children were born to unwed mothers (Robinson and Paikin 2001). Notwithstanding the increasing numbers of unwed mothers and the likely increases in incomplete certificates, state laws continue to do little to encourage full, accurate, informed, and timely birth records (Estin 2001, 1408). Legislative inaction may be traced to concerns about promoting nonmarital family relationships at the expense of marriages. But such concerns offer insufficient justification for the continuing gaps in birth record laws. If the birth certificate for an unwed mother is incomplete, the mother usually has no legal duty to notify the natural father of the birth and no legal duty to secure for the child a later designation of legal paternity when it is available. Birth certificates may be amended later, but changes that add the natural father are not mandated, and later governmental inquiries into missing information often are not very searching or are haphazard, if they occur at all. Furthermore, when an unwed natural mother places her child for adoption shortly after birth, often she is not required to identify the natural father (or the suspects) by name (confidentially). Her account of the natural father's disinterest, abandonment, failure of support, and the like, even when not in an affidavit or when incredible, is usually taken at face value. Finally, when an unwed natural mother maintains sole custody of a child with no designation of legal paternity, usually she is not encouraged by government to complete the birth certificate or otherwise identify the father, unless she later seeks certain forms of financial assistance from the government on behalf of her child.

What were the likely birth certificate procedures used if the woman in the song gave birth to her child in the United States? If she was married to the Other Man, he may have been named as the father, whether or not he knew of the circumstances of the pregnancy or that he was not genetically tied, he was deceived by his wife about genetic ties, he encouraged her to seek out the Lonely Boy, or he knew the prevailing laws on paternity presumptions and on the standards for rebuttal.

If the mother was not married to the Other Man, he may have been named as father, again whether or not he knew about genetic ties, any deception, the Lonely Boy, or the prevailing laws on paternity. Such a designation may have been prompted by his preconception or postconception promise to father his girlfriend's later-born child. But it need not. If he was not named, the rationales may have included maternal disinclination, his unwillingness to rear a child in the absence of genetic ties, or his belief (perhaps correct) that only natural fathers should be designated (with adoption available later to other men wishing to father).

When the birth certificate names a father, it is often the first but not the last legal paternity designation. Multiple and inconsistent legal paternity designations may be made for a single child. For example, although a birth certificate may designate the husband as the "presumed" father, the mother, the husband, the natural father, or the child may have some standing in a later court proceeding to challenge this presumption. And, though a birth certificate and an order in a marriage dissolution proceeding may designate a married couple as parents, these designations may be challenged in a later paternity action brought by the child or perhaps by an alleged natural father, as neither was party to the earlier proceedings. In a West Virginia case, a birth certificate that did not name the father was followed by inconsistent legal paternity designations accomplished through a notarized paternity acknowledgment, an amended birth certificate, a child support case finding, and another child support case finding (*State ex rel. W.Va. Dep't of Health* 2000).

Better legal paternity designations would follow if more complete, informed, and accurate birth records shortly after birth were promoted by laws requiring that expectant mothers, new mothers, and others who are specially interested (including husbands and boyfriends) receive better information about the legal consequences of birth. For example, professionals providing childbirth services could be required to pass on information to all women, and perhaps others in attendance, about the relevant state laws on paternity, including the laws on prebirth parental responsibilities, presumed fatherhood, the support obligations of unwed men, and the duties of natural fathers married to other women (Resnick, Wartenberg, and Brewer 1994, 298–99). If possible, information should be distributed some significant time before birth to promote informed planning and more deliberate and informed birth certificates. Services such as counseling, legal representation, and scientific testing should be provided to those in need.

Laws should also promote more conclusive legal paternity designations, even if they occur some time after birth. Thus the state could usually require periodic inquiry (by state agents, such as record keepers, or by hospital personnel) into the legal paternity of a child whose birth record, without explanation, lacks the name of a male parent. These inquiries, at least, should involve the dissemination of (additional) information on legal paternity and on available governmental services. Legal paternity inquiries and designations should not always be encouraged, however, such as for births that seemingly result from male criminal sexual assaults.

Lawmakers also should consider the circumstances appropriate for revived legal paternity. Here, genetic ties would give certain men a second chance to develop an "enduring" parent-child relationship. Unlike retroactive legal paternity, in which paternity based on genetics is established long after birth but relates back in time to the date of birth (often for child support purposes), revived paternity rights would be based, at least in part, on genetics but would not relate back. Revived rights should be especially considered for those rare cases of children who have no legal or actual parents and would benefit from "enduring" relationships with their natural fathers, though other prospective fathers (such as adopters) might also be available. Consider, for example, what should happen if the woman in the song were unmarried and died shortly after childbirth and after encountering again the Lonely Boy, and the Other Man had no interest in parenting. Such revived paternity rights would then allow other blood relatives the chance to bond (not inconsequential, given, for example, recent grandparent visitation initiatives).

These suggested reforms do not address the substantive law differences among U.S. states on matters of legal paternity. In all likelihood, the absence of unifying federal constitutional law standards will continue, as will significant differences between states in such areas as paternity law presumptions, state constitutional law recognitions of parental rights, and the legal treatment of deceitful acts by mothers involving men's actual or potential genetic ties to children. Nevertheless, procedural law reforms directed at birth certificate designations do seem appropriate for lawmakers in the U.S. Congress. Thus, when pondering state-to-state procedural law reforms involving legal paternity, Congress should consider the possibility of comprehensive regulation by congressional certification processes for all births in the United States. Even well-grounded state procedural law initiatives can only do so much. Although states are unlikely to unify on substance in the foreseeable future, certainty and much other good would flow from uniform federal statutory procedures on the mechanisms for designating legal paternity.

Either federal or state paternity procedure reforms carry hard-to-read price tags. The story told in the Heart song illustrates the difficult social policy issues. Requirements prompting new or additional governmental investigations into procreational activities would undercut the freedoms enjoyed today by many women regarding male involvement in their children's lives. The federal constitutional informational privacy, procreational, and child-rearing rights of women must be respected. Yet there seemingly are also parental opportunity interests or child-rearing rights for at least some Lonely Boys, men genetically tied to the children born to women who are distanced from them. Where those interests or rights are lost, especially with little or no culpability on the part of the Lonely Boy, should he inevitably remain on the hook for possible child support? Should the assumption at birth of legal or actual parenthood by the Other Man foreclose not only the Lonely Boy's parental rights but also his possible support obligations? If so, should the government seek to ensure that the Other Man acts in an informed way?

Concerns about promoting designations of parentage only for heterosexual couples also arise. New laws need not require that all or most children have at least one male parent. A child born as a result of a rape or through artificial insemination by an anonymous donor may never have a male parent under law. Or, a child born to an unwed mother who has been artificially inseminated by an anonymous donor should in certain settings be recognized as having two female parents (as when two women have agreed to shared parenting). Birth certificate procedures should reflect these concerns.

The suggested reforms for legal paternity designations may still mean that some natural fathers will lose forever the opportunity to parent, through no fault of their own. But this is already happening far too frequently. Reforms may also result in some men with no genetic ties forever carrying legal paternity designations because of their earlier factual assumptions or their reliance on lies. And, it may mean that women will be less able to conceal the identity of natural fathers. These are significant costs. Nevertheless, our present birth certificate and other paternity designation procedures seem more costly. For children born in the United States, federal and state governments and most Americans have compelling interests in better assuring that correct and lasting legal paternity designations are made at birth.

Conclusion

State substantive law guidelines for paternity vary significantly, often differing even in a single state depending on context. These guidelines are implemented through a variety of state-controlled procedures, including birth certificates, paternity cases, court findings during marriage dissolutions, and paternity registrations. Not infrequently these procedures do not adequately promote the legitimate governmental and private interests in early, complete, accurate, informed, and conclusive legal paternity designations. Undesirable conduct by mothers or others can lead to successive legal paternity designations that are inconsistent, fortuitous, and inconclusive. Currently there are too many unfair foreclosures of paternal interests and rights and too many unfair assignments of paternal responsibilities, because of unnecessary "procedural quirks, complications and limitations" (*Gunn v. Cavanaugh* 1965).

American legal paternity procedures are fundamentally flawed. Perhaps they encourage a woman who wants a child to make "love" with a "lonely boy," even though she knows that she will abandon him because she is in love with "another man" (who may not know of her actions), and even though she might later pursue the boy for child support. Contemporary laws also encourage a Lonely Boy who is interested in his genetic ties to a child to seek out, if not stalk, his former lover in order to learn of any pregnancy or birth. Where such an inquiry is not undertaken or is unsuccessful and his parental rights are lost, state laws nevertheless may require this same man to provide child support long after any real chance has passed for him to establish an enduring parent-child relationship. Furthermore, contemporary laws sometimes allow the Other Man, who could not give the woman the "one little thing" she desired, to disestablish or lose legal paternity long after he actually began to father, even when the child's best interests are not promoted.

Questions raised by the song linger. While some may be unanswerable by lawmakers, many are not. American paternity law reforms are long overdue. As changes are contemplated, serious attention should be given to the possible federalization of birth certificate procedures for children born in the United States through consensual sexual intercourse. At the least, individual states should reform their legal paternity procedures so that legal fatherhood at the time of a child's birth is more often conclusively and accurately established immediately after the birth.

ACKNOWLEDGMENTS

This chapter draws significantly from, and expands on, my earlier works, including "Designating Male Parents at Birth" (*University of Michigan Journal of Law Reform* 26 [1993]: 573–92), concluding that current designations of a child's male parentage at the time of birth often are made inconsistently, fortuitously, inconclusively, and without involving all interested parties; "Pregnant Dads: The Crimes and Other Misconduct of Expectant Fathers" (*Oregon Law Review* 72 [1993]: 901–18), urging more discussion of the legal duties of expectant dads; "Abortions of the Parental Prerogatives of Unwed Natural Fathers: Deterring Host Paternity" (*Oklahoma Law Review* 53 [2000]: 345–87), suggesting how governments may better safeguard the parenthood opportunities of unwed natural fathers; "Old-Fashioned Pregnancy, Newly Fashioned Paternity" (*Syracuse Law Review* 53 [2003]: 57–86), recommending additional procedural law protections for natural fathers; "Participation of Unwed Biological Fathers in Newborn Adoptions: Achieving Substantive and Procedural Fairness" (*Journal of Law and Family Studies* 5 [2003]: 223–37), suggesting fairer procedures during newborn adoptions; and "Federalizing Birth Certificate Procedures" (*Brandeis Law Journal* 42 [2003]: 105–27), urging congressional action.

Lyrics from the song "All I Want to Do Is Make Love to You," by Lange, are published by Zomba Music Publisher, Ltd. Used by permission.

BIBLIOGRAPHY

Caban v. Mohammed. 1979. 441 U.S. 380, 397.
Estin, A. L. 2001. Ordinary cohabitation. *Notre Dame Law Review* 76:1381–1408.
Glennon, T. 2000. Somebody's child: Evaluating the erosion of the marital presumptions of paternity. *West Virginia Law Review* 102:547–605.
Gunn v. Cavanaugh. 1965. 391 S.W.2d 723, 727 (Tex.).
Kaplan, D. S. 2000. Why truth is not a defense in paternity actions. *Texas Journal of Women and the Law* 10:69–81.
Lehr v. Robertson. 1983. 463 U.S. 248, 262.
Michael H. v. Gerald D. 1989. 491 U.S. 110, 115.
Nguyen v. INS. 2001. 533 U.S. 53, 62–63.
Resnick, M. D., E. Wartenberg, and R. Brewer. 1994. The fate of the non-marital child: A challenge to the health system. *Journal of Community Health* 19:285–99.
Robinson, B., and S. Paikin. 2001. Who is daddy? A case for the Uniform Parentage Act (2001). *Delaware Lawyer* 19:23–27.
State ex rel. W.Va. Dep't of Health and Human Resources. 2000. 531 S.E.2d 669 (W.Va.).
United States Commission on Interstate Child Support. 1992. *Supporting Our Children: A Blueprint for Reform.* Washington, DC: The Commission.

CHAPTER TEN

Disestablishment Suits

Daddy No More?

Mary Anderlik Majumder, J.D., Ph.D.

The first wave of DNA-based identity testing coincided with an aggressive program of paternity establishment for nonmarital children receiving federal welfare benefits. Although the launch of testing in this environment was a significant development, the public purposes behind testing were well understood, the rules for testing were relatively clear, and the program was consistent with long-standing commitments to establishing family relationships and promoting responsibility. The second wave of testing is being driven by private interests, the rules for testing are unclear, and the genetic test results increasingly have the effect of disrupting or "disestablishing" parent-child relationships and triggering demands for the elimination of responsibility. Courts and state legislatures are searching for ways to reconcile the competing rights and interests. So far, there is little evidence of consensus.

The current problems would not exist were it not for advances in science and technology. The Human Genome Project has accelerated the development of techniques for inexpensive, efficient analysis of regions of DNA and comparison of genetic profiles. Scientists and engineers are constantly refining those techniques, meaning that testing is becoming ever faster, cheaper, and more widely available. Even with existing technologies, analysis can be performed on DNA extracted from almost any biological material. Testing at one time required a blood draw, but many laboratories now offer testing with sample collection by mail (referred to as "mail order," "home," or "do-it-yourself" testing) using cheek swabs. The Human Genome Project has also increased interest in genetic identity as an aspect of health care.

Beyond this, the emphasis on genetic identity has reinforced the view that biological relationship and parental status are tightly linked. The tests used to prove biological paternity can also be used to disprove biological paternity. Given the growing influence of genetic thinking and "genetic essentialism," it is easy to slide into the view that genetic contribution is the essence of family and fatherhood (Nelkin and Lindee 1995).

Finally, DNA-based identity testing has now become part of the culture, with paternity testing a staple of talk shows and daytime and prime-time dramas (Stanley 2002). Media attention and the marketing efforts of laboratories have contributed to demand for testing by sowing suspicion about paternity and fidelity *and* suggesting that testing is a natural and acceptable response to suspicion.

Reliable evidence concerning the extent of misidentified paternity in the general population is not available. There are some indications that the incidence may be surprisingly high (Anderlik 2003). Historically, the law favored stability over accuracy in attribution of paternity, but that was before definitive proof of paternity or nonpaternity was possible. Science and technology have changed the circumstances. Should the law change as well?

A Review of the Legal Landscape

The stories of men such as Gerald Miscovich (*Miscovich v. Miscovich* 1997), Dennis Caron (*Caron v. Manfresca* 1999), and Morgan Wise (*Wise v. Fryar* 2001) have been the catalysts for debate on a husband's power to terminate legal responsibility—to "disestablish" paternity—in cases where testing reveals or confirms the absence of biological relationship. Cases in which men attempt to end child support obligations assumed in connection with a voluntary acknowledgment of paternity raise a similar set of issues. Both kinds of cases create concerns about the psychological, emotional, and financial welfare of the children and adults involved as well as concerns about fairness. Further, the financial importance of parentage determination does not end with child support; social security, health insurance, survivors' benefits, military benefits, and inheritance rights hang in the balance. There are also broader social policy concerns when families are destabilized, and not only when the disappearance from the scene of a presumed or acknowledged father affects the public purse. The men bringing delayed disestablishment suits have often been unsuccessful in the courts, but these losses have sometimes translated into victories in the legislature.

A Complex Legal Background

There is a long and convoluted history behind the presumption that a husband is the legal father of the children born to his wife during their marriage, commonly referred to as the "marital presumption" or "presumption of legitimacy," and with advances in testing the application of the presumption has become a matter of increasing perplexity. Historically, the marital presumption was perhaps best characterized as a rule of evidence. A presumption favors a particular inference about underlying facts. Before the development of blood tests capable of excluding biological relationship, marital status was a reasonable proxy for biological relationship in circumstances in which a man's status as progenitor could seldom be established with certainty. If the husband's paternity was a physical impossibility—that is, in cases of absence or impotence or sterility—the marital presumption either did not apply or could be rebutted by this evidence bearing on the facts of conception.

Yet that was not the whole story. The courts developed supplemental rules affecting the ability to bring a lawsuit and the admissibility of evidence, rules that blocked challenges to legitimacy even in cases where the biological fatherhood of a man other than the husband was all but certain. Hence, other social policy considerations, such as protecting the institution of marriage or the welfare of children, have long played a role in the application of the marital presumption. With the emergence of human leukocyte antigen testing and then genetic testing, some courts in effect "converted" the presumption into a substantive rule of law intended to protect the integrity of the marital family and secure the welfare of children. In other words, within certain parameters, these courts began to treat the presumption as a principle tying legal fatherhood to social relationship, versus a provisional assignment of legal fatherhood based on assumed biological relationship.

The process of evolution has, unfortunately, left the law in many states with distinctions that make little sense, regardless of the rationale. For example, in keeping with the traditional formulations removing cases of physical impossibility from the scope of the marital presumption, California's "conclusive presumption" operates only if husband and wife are cohabiting and the husband is not impotent or sterile (Cal. Family Code § 7540). A related statutory provision allows for challenges based on blood tests, but only within a two-year window from the child's birth (Cal. Family Code § 7541). Hence medical testing five or ten years after birth could translate into a disestablishment suit if it revealed that the husband could not have been the biological father because he was sterile, but not if it revealed the impossibility of biological fatherhood on some other basis. There is little logic here. If marriage with cohabitation matters in paternity determination as a proxy for biological paternity, then blood test evidence of the husband's exclusion as a biological father, like evidence of impotence or sterility, should remove the case from the scope of the presumption. If marriage with cohabitation matters in paternity determination for social policy reasons because it suggests the existence of a stable family unit, then the same restrictions should apply to all efforts to disestablish the husband as legal father.

In addition, in many states, statutory provisions that relate to presumptions of paternity and actions to establish the existence or nonexistence of paternity, standing to invoke or challenge presumptions, time limits on challenges, and genetic testing have been drawn from diverse sources over time and are lodged in multiple sections of the family law code or title or in the law of trusts and estates. For example, Florida law presents a confusing jumble of presumptions and rules relating to obligations of support derived from the common law and from statutory procedures for establishment of paternity that can be traced back to a bastardy law enacted in 1828 (Altenbernd 1999). It is not always clear how these provisions are to be reconciled.

Another source of complexity is the interplay between family law and the rules of civil procedure that govern court proceedings generally. In many disestablishment cases, a man's status as legal father has been created or affirmed by a judgment or order, typically at the conclusion of a divorce or paternity proceeding. Usually the rules will specify that a motion to reopen a judgment due to mistake or newly discovered evidence must be filed within a certain number of years or a "reasonable" period of time. There is controversy over whether this kind of limit applies to newly available genetic evidence of nonpaternity (*Tandra S. v. Tyrone W.* 1994; *Langston v. Riffe* 2000). Also, exceptions to time limits are generally made in cases involving fraud. The question then becomes how strict a standard to employ. Is a woman's silence or reassurance concerning paternity the kind of fraud that should support reopening of a judgment? The policy arguments supporting a standard that demands more than this for reopening of a judgment would include the state interest in finality of judgments. Finality may advance child welfare as well as efficiency in the administration of the child welfare system. At the same time, a strict standard may "invite suspicion and distrust and essentially require all purported fathers, upon divorce or separation, to accuse their spouses or partners of infidelity by demanding proof of paternity" in the context of the proceeding (*Smith v. Dep't of Human Resources* 1997). Of course, some increase in suspicion and distrust may be tolerable if early establishment of biological identity is important.

In addition to the doctrine of *res judicata*, courts may invoke a number of equitable doctrines to change the outcome in paternity cases. As the term suggests, equitable doctrines are principles that allow judges to ignore or adjust the usual legal rules if strict application would work an injustice. One approach to achieving equity is to prevent or "estop" a person from asserting a legal right. In disestablishment cases, the doctrine of equitable estoppel can enter the picture in a number of ways. For example, a man may be estopped from disavowing paternity, or he may claim the benefit of estoppel in preserving the status of father against a wife or girlfriend denying a father-child relationship she formerly asserted. For an estoppel argument to succeed, an individual must generally show that another party engaged in a course of conduct inviting his or her reliance and that some detriment to the individual—or in a paternity case, to a dependent child—resulted or would result. So, for example, a man might be estopped (prevented) from disavowing paternity if he represented the child to others as his own and the child relied on the explicit or implicit representation of paternity in treating the man as father, offering him love and affection and looking to him for financial and emotional support (*Clevenger v. Clevenger* 1961). Courts seem most ready to estop a presumed, acknowledged, or adjudicated father from asserting nonpaternity if the man knew or should have known that he was not the biological father much earlier in time and failed to act, and if the alleged detrimental reliance is at least in part financial, such as where there is reason to believe that another man would have been pursued for support had the presumed or acknowledged or adjudicated father taken himself out of the way (*Rubright v. Arnold* 1999; *B.E.B. v. R.L.B.* 1999; *State v. Kovac* 1999; *In re Marriage of A.J.N. & J.M.N.* 1987).

Some commentators urge courts to consider possible gender bias as they exercise their equitable powers. When women advance estoppel arguments against husbands and others on behalf of children, they stand a good chance of losing. Men have generally been successful with estoppel arguments when women seek to oust them from relationships with children. In these cases, there may be a tendency to label the men dupes and the women schemers. This conscious or subconscious form of stereotyping can result in inequitable application of the doctrine of estoppel (Glennon 2000, 2001).

Finally, presumptions and other rules affecting parentage determination may impinge on constitutional rights. Usually, challenges to state paternity laws are based on the due process or equal protection clauses of the U.S. Constitution, or parallel provisions in a state constitution. One common scenario involves a contest between a presumed father and an alleged biological father, in which establishment of the paternity of the latter amounts to disestablishment of the former. The most famous case of this nature is *Michael H. v. Gerald D.* (1989). *Michael H.* was decided by the U.S. Supreme Court in 1989. At issue in *Michael H.* was California's conclusive presumption of paternity. A man who had obtained proof of his biological paternity through genetic testing and had taken steps to develop a parent-child relationship claimed that the law violated his constitutional due process rights because it gave him no opportunity to make his case for fatherhood. A fractured Supreme Court upheld the California law.

As late as the 1970s, the right to bring an action for establishment of paternity in Florida was limited to unmarried women. A married woman who wished to establish the paternity of a man not her husband challenged this restriction. The Florida Supreme Court, in *Gammon v. Cobb* (1976), noted the potential for "anomalous" situations in which "the reputed father of an illegitimate child born to his wife can attack the child's parentage and be relieved of the obligation to support the child, but at the same time the wife may not maintain a suit to compel the putative or natural father to provide support for the child." The court ruled that the portion of the law limiting actions to unmarried women was unconstitutional. Laws that allow male defendants, but no one else, to introduce new "scientific evidence" at any time may also present equal protection problems.

A Typology of Contemporary Responses

A basic value question underlying much of the policy debate on parentage determination is, to what degree should biology be controlling in the formation of families and, more particularly, the award of the rights and responsibilities of parenthood? The possible responses can be organized in terms of four positions. I will first sketch each position as an "ideal type" and then show how the position figures in legal rhetoric and reality.

Biological imperative. For those who adopt this position, legal rules and the outcomes are, or ought to be, dictated by biology. Parenthood, and the rights and responsibilities associated with parent-child relationships, are seen as necessarily grounded in and flowing out of biological relationships. This is an ancient and still highly influential way of thinking about the family. On the one hand, this position may reflect a view that biological connection itself creates a bond between parent and child so strong that separation is virtually unendurable, so powerful that the biological parent is compelled to subordinate his or her own interests to those of the child. Therefore, biological matching of parent and child must, in some sense, advance the welfare of the child, because the parent known or revealed as having a mere social connection to the child will inevitably fail to fulfill the child's deepest needs. This view may be fostered and strengthened by the increasing attention to genes and genetics in the media. On the other hand, the biological imperative may be viewed solely in terms of financial responsibility. In the context of contemporary U.S. social institutions, engaging in activity that may produce a child creates a duty to pay to support any child resulting from that activity.

The idea of a biological imperative seems to exert considerable influence on some state legislators—legislators who have translated the rhetoric of fathers' (or men's) rights groups into bills and statutes. Cases in which men are refused release from obligations to children in the face of genetic test results excluding them as biological fathers have prompted vigorous advocacy by these groups. Those within the fathers' rights movement tend to view family law through the lens of criminal law. The crusade to free men of unwanted paternity in such cases is presented as a kind of "Innocence Project" (Citizens against Paternity Fraud 2005; Quinn 2001). It is common to find the issue framed as one of justice or fairness, in the sense that evidence admissible to "convict" should also be available to "exonerate." Anger over the outcomes in particular cases has fueled fierce lobbying for laws to correct the perceived injustices. For example, in 2000, following the uproar over the treatment of Dennis Caron (*Caron v. Manfresca* 1999), Ohio passed a law requiring relief from a child support order at any time following proof of biological exclusion and opening the door for lawsuits to recover child support already paid from mothers or biological fathers (Ohio H.B. 242, 1999). A marriage to the mother or any admission or acknowledgment of paternity is irrelevant under the Ohio law, if the man was not aware of his nonpaternity at the time. The law includes a declaration that the man has a "substantive right" to relief. Yet Ohio and other states that have these kinds of laws are not necessarily consistent in their adherence to the biological imperative. Under these laws, the women and children affected, and the biological father, may have no right to challenge the status of a presumed father who wishes to continue a legal relationship.

Others have advocated mandatory genetic testing at birth or at another key juncture such as divorce. This may seem far from feasible, but the approach is being taken seriously in some quarters. In the course of oral argument for a disestablishment case involving the presumed father of a marital child, a justice on the Florida Supreme Court queried, "Are we really saying . . . in the future DNA testing will have to be part of every divorce or custody hearing?" (Follick 2000, 6). At least one Florida legislator thought the answer was yes. House Bill 73, prefiled in 2001 but withdrawn before introduction, would have required DNA paternity testing in all divorce and child support proceedings (Florida H.B. 73, 2001).

In disestablishment cases decided to date, the biological imperative position shows up most frequently in concurring or dissenting opinions, suggesting that it is somewhat idiosyncratic among judges. Concurring in part and dissenting in part in a disestablishment case, a justice on the Alabama Supreme Court wrote:

> While debate continues over the relative influences of heredity and environment, one thing is clear—the mystic bonds of blood are strong. The strength of these bonds is illustrated in various ways and is observable in ordinary experience. A familiar example is that of adopted children who are nurtured to maturity by exemplary adoptive parents, but, nevertheless, ultimately feel compelled to seek out their biological parents . . . A strong sense of personal identity is an asset, and personal identity derives in large measure from knowledge of, and association with, individuals of biological kinship (*Ex parte Jenkins* 1998).

Allied to this position are statements that science promises truth about fatherhood. For example, in his dissent in the *Michael H.* case, U.S. Supreme Court Justice William J. Brennan wrote that California law "stubbornly" insisted on labeling the mother's husband "father" in the face of evidence showing a 98 percent probability to the contrary (*Michael H. v. Gerald D.* 1989). And in a decision striking down a state statute denying a putative biological father his day in court as unconstitutional, the Texas Supreme Court expressed the view that the state's interest in minimizing familial disruptions may have "had merit in an earlier era when the true biological father could not be established with near certainty and when illegitimacy carried a significant legal and social stigma," but no longer (*In re J.W.T.* 1994).

Biological presumption. For those who adopt this position, all other things being equal, biology controls. In other words, claims based on biology may sometimes be limited to accommodate important individual rights and interests (child or adult) or to serve the interests of society, but the burden of proof is clearly on the one arguing for a departure from biology. By making biology nearly, but not quite, controlling, it is possible to preserve some of the benefits associated with having a "bright line" rule, such as efficiency in decision making, with fewer cases going to the courts and faster resolution when they do. Also, if the belief that genetically related adults are likely to be better nurturers of children than other adults has any truth to it, there is reason to favor biology. Exceptions will be made only to avoid demonstrably bad results or serious violations of rights in particular cases. By allowing some room for rights and other types of claims not based in biology, this position is in line with two broader trends in public policy concerning the family. First, intention has become increasingly important in family law, as reflected in cases dealing with assisted reproduction. Second, in areas of law affecting children, there has been a movement to make the best interests of the child the standard for decision making, despite worries that the best interests standard is vague and open to bias in application.

The influence of this position on legislators can be detected in "hybrid" approaches that make biology determinative for a limited period of time. Under the revised Uniform Parentage Act of 2000 (UPA), as amended in 2002, a proceeding to adjudicate parentage for a child with a presumed father may be commenced within two years after birth, but not thereafter (UPA § 607). There is also a two-year window for challenges to voluntary acknowledgments of paternity, including any challenge brought by an acknowledged father on the basis of "fraud, duress, or material mistake of fact" once a sixty-day rescission period has passed (UPA §§ 308, 309, 609). A child is not bound by a determination of parentage under the act unless the outcome is supported by genetic test results or the child is represented in the proceeding (UPA § 637).

Even within the two-year window, a court is authorized to deny a request for genetic testing when there is a presumed father if (1) the conduct of the mother or presumed father estops that party from denying parentage and (2) disproving the relationship would be inequitable (UPA §§ 608, 609[c]). The model law provides that, in making its determination, the court "shall consider" the best interests of the child, to include, among other things, the length of time elapsed since the presumed father was placed on notice that he might not be the genetic father, the length of time the presumed father occupied the role of father, the facts surrounding the discovery of possible nonpaternity, the nature of the father-child relationship, the child's age, the potential harm to the child, and the potential for establishing the paternity of another man. In such a case, a guardian *ad litem* must be appointed to represent the child. However, the standard for a denial of testing is a high one—it must be based on "clear and convincing" evidence. Fundamentally, fathering is viewed as a biological event, and granting or imposing parental status based on social relationship rather than biology is exceptional. Still, the child's interest in security and the state's interest in definitively establishing responsibility eclipse biology with the passage of time.

The American Law Institute (ALI) takes a somewhat similar approach to these issues in its *Principles of the Law of Family Dissolution* (American Law Institute 2002). The ALI principles are concerned with custody decisions and determinations of child support obligations rather than with parentage determinations per se. Also, it is important to note that the principles are not a model law but rather a summary and guide founded on a review of existing state law. In keeping with an emphasis on the functional components of parenting, the definition of *parent* includes not only the persons defined as parents under other state law but also a "parent by estoppel," such as an individual who had a reasonable, good-faith belief that he was the child's father, lived with the child, and fully accepted the responsibilities of parenthood for at least two years (ALI 2002, § 2.03). In deciding whether to impose a support obligation on a person who is not a legal parent, courts are directed to consider factors such as how the person and the child have acted toward each other, whether the relationship supplanted the child's opportunity to develop a relationship with an absent parent, and whether the child otherwise has two parents who are able and available to discharge obligations of support (ALI 2002, § 3.03). Compared with the UPA, the ALI principles represent a loosening of the hold of biology, a movement toward the position of biological relevance with its emphasis on social relationships.

Biological relevance. Relevance means that biology counts—along with other factors. It is entitled to some weight, but it is not the whole story, or maybe even the most important part of the story. The view that biological relationship is the exclusive determinant or essence of the parent-child relationship has never been without challenge. The Romans used the term *alumnus* to designate an abandoned child taken in and raised by a biological stranger. Inscriptions establish that such children were cherished, and this arrangement could be cited as a model of the kind of love and kindness characteristic of the highest forms of human relationship (Murray 1996). A contemporary parallel would be the celebration of "psychological parenting." According to Goldstein and colleagues, "for the child, the physical realities of his conception and birth are not the direct cause of his emotional attachment. This attachment results from day-to-day attention to his needs for physical care, nourishment, comfort, affection, and stimulation" (Goldstein, Freud, and Solnit 1979, 17). A lessening of the emphasis on the biological tie may also reflect greater comfort with the idea that, through their relationships with children, presumed fathers may incur responsibilities that continue even after the biological basis for the relationship is revealed as an illusion. Although law cannot force men to continue as psychological parents, it might foster and reinforce an expectation that bonds of affection and care nourished over time will sustain the relationship once the initial shock of a finding of biological exclusion has passed.

In re Cheryl, decided by the Supreme Judicial Court of Massachusetts in 2001, sits somewhere between biological presumption and biological relevance. A man who became a legal father by means of a voluntary acknowledgment moved to set aside the judgment based on genetic tests obtained five years later. The court ruled against him, in the light of his failure to exercise his right to genetic testing before acknowledgment, evidence of the development of a father-child relationship, and his persistence in the relationship even after he had reason to suspect an absence of biological connection. The court affirmed the public interest in the finality of paternity judgments, citing the best interests of the child. Further, in the best interests analysis, the court stressed stability and continuity. The court was careful to note the empirical foundation for this weighting of factors: "Social science data and literature overwhelmingly establish that children benefit psychologically, socially, educationally and in other ways from stable and predictable parental relationships . . . This holds true even where the father is a noncustodial parent . . . , or where the stable relationship is with an individual not genetically linked to the child" (*In re Cheryl* 2001). Yet the court did not declare biology irrelevant. Noting the anomaly of continuing a legal status and responsibility begun solely on the basis of an asserted biological connection in the face of proof of its absence, the court stated that a different result might be not only appropriate but mandated if a man challenged a paternity judgment promptly on obtaining information raising questions about genetic ties to the child.

Intermediate positions such as biological presumption and biological relevance allow for considerable flexibility and may be associated with greater receptivity to nonexclusive family structures. In Louisiana, cases brought by marital children seeking benefits resting on recognition of the paternity of their extramarital biological fathers opened the door to a variety of actions, eroding the "fiction" that the legal father was the only father (*Smith v. Cole* 1989). But the legal or presumed father did not simply go away. The Louisiana courts recognize the potential for continuing responsibilities and rights, if no disavowal is made by the man within the statutorily prescribed period, and if continuing the legal relationship in some form accords with the best interests of the child.

Judgment is context-specific. For example, in *Geen v. Geen* (1995), the legal father and primary custodial parent retained that status even after testing proved that another man, who eventually married the mother, was the biological father, and even after the mother and her new husband sought custody. The decision rested on a best interests analysis that gave most weight to psychological parenthood: "Geen has provided Ryan with a stable, wholesome environment, a permanent custodial home, and a close and continuing, loving relationship since Ryan's birth, always putting Ryan's interest above his own. He has fed him, dressed him, bathed him, provided medical care, and selected a school, after thoroughly investigating that school." The court also considered it important that Geen "encouraged and facilitated a close and continuing relationship between Ryan and his other two parents" (*Geen v. Geen* 1995).

Biological indifference. Opposing the biological imperative is the position that biology is a matter of indifference. On this view, policy—and outcomes in particular cases—should be dictated by intention to parent, one's engagement in parenting behavior, considerations of child welfare, or social factors such as strengthening the institution of marriage. If biology is to be considered at all, it would be solely as a matter of convenience or as a factor in the analysis of the best interests of the child. For example, for pragmatic reasons, a society might decide that children should stay with birth parents unless and until some kind of dispute arises. In the event of dispute, the judge charged with assigning parental rights and responsibilities would ask which person would be the best parent, that is, the most nurturing, the most consistent presence, the best equipped financially to support the child, and so on. Biological relationship to the child would have no independent significance.

As might be expected, adoption of the position of biological indifference is rare in law. In his *Michael H.* opinion, Justice Antonin Scalia, faced with a line of U.S. Supreme Court cases recognizing fathers' rights in relation to nonmarital children, asserted that those rights arose from the "sanctity" of the "unitary family" rather than biological contribution. In 1993, an Ohio court ruled that a statute giving a putative biological father legal standing to establish paternity in relation to a child within an intact marital family violated the due process clause of the state constitution by infringing on the right to marital privacy and the right to raise children without state-authorized intrusion. The court found the state's interest in determining paternity strictly on the basis of genetics "at most insubstantial, if not completely nonexistent" (*Merkel v. Doe* 1993).

In Pennsylvania, courts have held that "no amount of evidence" can overcome the marital presumption if the family remains intact at the time the husband's paternity is challenged. The policy goal of preserving marriages trumps all other considerations (*Strauser v. Stahr* 1999). These courts have also been ready to apply the doctrine of estoppel to preserve father-child relationships, whether or not created within a marriage, based on a policy that "children should be secure in knowing who their parents are" (*Brinkley v. King* 1997). The victory of marriage or continuity and stability in parent-child relationships over biology is not secure, however. If it were, the Pennsylvania courts elevating marriage and continuity over biology would not label their legal rules "fictions." The Pennsylvania Supreme Court has suggested that truth must be sacrificed when biology is ignored in the service of the greater social good: "the presumption of paternity embodies the fiction that regardless of biology, the married people to whom the child was born are the parents; and the doctrine of estoppel embodies the fiction that, regardless of biology, in the absence of a marriage, the person who has cared for the child is the parent" (*Brinkley v. King* 1997).

A Return to the Best Interests of the Child

In a recent disestablishment case, the Colorado Supreme Court was called on to interpret statutory language directing judges to look at the weight of policy and logic in selecting among conflicting presumptions of paternity.

The magistrate hearing the case in the first instance had equated "logic" with scientific evidence of biological paternity. The Supreme Court suggested that a more complex understanding of paternity is required. According to the court's interpretation of Colorado law, the presumption of legal fatherhood based on genetic evidence of biological relationship is itself rebuttable, not by additional evidence bearing on biology but by evidence concerning the best interests of the child. Even marriage or family preservation count only insofar as these are shown to advance the best interests of children. As to the essence of parent-hood, the court remarked, "Perhaps, as King Solomon observed many centuries ago in a battle over parentage, the true parent is the one who can elevate the best interests of the child over his or her own best interests" (*N.A.H. v. S.L.S* 2000).

The best interests standard, for all the criticism it has faced, seems a good touchstone for decision making about disestablishment of paternity. All the positions described in the typology of responses have some basis in a desire to advance the welfare of children, and the topic seems worthy of further explo-ration in the context of disestablishment.

The Best Interests Analysis

Some elements are almost always considered as part of a best interests analysis, such as the need for permanence or stability in the life of a child and provision for material support. Theresa Glennon has noted the difficulties that attend attempts to assess the quality of relationships versus the use of more objective criteria (Glennon 2000). Unfortunately, there are no studies that track the effects of different decision rules or guidelines for parentage as-signment on child welfare. Those who endorse multiple fatherhood must ad-dress the concern that diffusion of responsibility will lead to neglect on the part of the parents and confusion on the part of the child.

Elements in the best interests analysis particularly relevant to the genetic testing context include identity formation and interests related to health or medical care. Some have put forward a concept of "genealogical bewilder-ment" to describe the negative psychological consequences of ignorance of one's origins. However, the primary evidence for such a phenomenon seems to be literary (e.g., the Oedipal myth and the story of the Ugly Duckling) and anecdotal (Sants 1964). Still, the growing trend of open adoption seems trace-able, in part, to a recognition that there are benefits to children in knowing about and perhaps developing social relationships with biological parents and other kin. A sense of connection to an ethnic or cultural heritage is also increasingly recognized as important in the adoption context.

Courts may be more inclined to recognize an interest in an accurate family medical history than an abstract "right to know" one's origins. In one case, a court dispensed with the medical argument by noting that the alleged biological father had agreed to share his medical history regardless of the outcome of the paternity proceeding (*D.B.S. v. M.S.* 1995). Still, a few courts have cited a child's right to know the truth of her parentage for psychological and medical reasons as a significant consideration in their decision making. For example, a Connecticut court stated that, if paternity was not addressed at the time of the proceeding, it could "be raised to a devastating effect at some later point in the child's life" (*In re Jacqueline S.* 2001).

Glennon offers an Oklahoma statute as a model for its guidance on best interests analysis. The Oklahoma law "looks to readily identifiable factors, such as the child's age and residence with the alleged parent" and hence "gives courts a more easily administrable guideline and prevents courts from having to engage in more detailed, time-consuming, and ultimately confounding inquiries into the 'strength' of the parent-child bond" (Glennon 2001, 275). Glennon favors tailoring time limits and restrictions on disestablishment of paternity to child welfare. Her argument is reproduced here because it addresses some of the concerns about fairness raised by fathers' rights groups:

> While some individuals are innocent victims of deceptive partners, adults are aware of the high incidence of infidelity and only they, not the children, are able to act to ensure that the biological ties they may deem essential are present . . . The law should discourage adults from treating children they have parented as expendable when their adult relationships fall apart. It is adults who can and should absorb the pain of betrayal rather than inflict additional betrayal on the involved children (Glennon 2001, 281–82).

Fathers' rights advocates may have a stronger case when they assert the unfairness of holding a man liable for financial support but give him no protected interest in the opportunity to develop a relationship with a child. If the notion of fatherhood as necessarily an *exclusive* status is abandoned in nontraditional family situations, it becomes easier to join responsibilities with at least some correlative rights.

The assumptions underlying a policy decision to adopt a (more or less) conclusive presumption that the husband of the mother of a child is the child's progenitor and sole socially recognized, rights- and responsibility-bearing legal father include the following:

- A man can function as a good parent, even if a question has been raised about his genetic connection to a child;
- A marriage can survive the shock of an allegation of infidelity relatively intact;
- Social relationships are more important contributors to well-being than genetic relationships—for example, having an intact family is more important for child well-being than having an accurate understanding of genetic origins; but
- It is important to preserve the appearance of a family unit in which genetic and social relationships are aligned, and secrecy, or the suppression of information about (the absence of) genetic connection, may be required for a man to function as a good parent and/or for a marriage to survive.

The last assumption seems particularly difficult to sustain, given the increasing prevalence of blended families. Culturally, the blended family is less of an oddity than it was in the past, and hence social isolation or rejection is unlikely to result from acknowledgment of familial complexity in the area of biological and social relationships. Further, some studies on assisted reproduction have found that openness about a father's lack of biological connection to a child is associated with better outcomes, although there are inherent difficulties with studies of secrecy. The plurality opinion in *Michael H. v. Gerald D.* (1989) invoked "nature itself" to rule out the option of dual paternity. Interestingly, anthropologists have identified sixteen societies in South America marked by a belief in "partible paternity," that is, "the conviction that it is possible, even necessary, for a child to have more than one biological father" (*Economist* 1999). In one disestablishment case involving four psychologists, the final assessment was that the happy, well-adjusted child at the center of the dispute saw both his presumed father and his alleged biological father as "dad" (*D.B.S. v. M.S.* 1995).

Although the idea of multiple biological paternity may be at odds with science, short of some tricky genetic engineering, multiple fatherhood may make good social sense. Abandonment of the exclusive status model would free courts to conduct more nuanced best interests analyses. For example, a judge could conclude that genetic testing to clarify biological relationships is in the best interests of the child, as a means of averting harm from confusion or distress about identity and for medical reasons, without necessarily depriving a man who has had and wishes to continue a social relationship with the child of the title of father. At the conclusion of the testing process, if a new biological relationship were to be confirmed, the child would have two fathers, a legal father determined by criteria similar to those found in the Oklahoma law (likely the man with the established social relationship) and a biological father. The legal parents could be charged with determining the extent of any relationships with willing biological fathers or extended biological families in keeping with the best interests of the child. This would help guard against a problematic diffusion of responsibility. In unusual cases with circumstances suggesting that knowledge of a divide in fatherhood, or the identity of a biological father, might be harmful to a child, a best interests–based approach would give a judge discretion to deny testing.

Mandatory involvement of a guardian *ad litem* is another means of protecting the interests of children on a case-by-case basis, in the absence of bright line rules well-supported by the results of research concerning child welfare. Substantively, the best interests analysis should be expanded to recognize the greater potential for harm if there are multiple children in a family. Several courts have recognized the importance of ties to siblings, as well as extended family. Unfortunately, it is not unheard of for a man to terminate, or attempt to terminate, ties with a child while continuing visitation with siblings confirmed to be his biological offspring. This seems a recipe for disaster.

What the Law Can and Cannot Do

Anger and a desire to strike back at the women involved have clearly been significant factors in the fathers' rights movement, and the same complex of emotions may motivate some disestablishment suits. The Web site for the group Citizens against Paternity Fraud is the most emphatic in this regard; the Web site compares paternity fraud to rape and includes a "Hall of Paternity Fraud Victims" (www.paternityfraud.com). In media interviews and documents filed with courts, the men challenging court orders often say they do not necessarily want to discontinue support for a child (Brady 2001). Rather, they want to end the legal obligation to pay child support that might flow to the women who deceived them in two ways: by cheating on them and by lying to them about a child's paternity.

In some cases the insult seems fresh; in others, long-simmering suspicions, perhaps suppressed or contained in the interests of maintaining a valued relationship with a child, prompt action when a request is lodged for increased child support or the man starts another family. The cynical interpretation is that fatherhood is embraced unless and until it becomes inconvenient. More charitably, financial or other competing interests fuel resentment against the mother and the legal system for its imposition of responsibilities. The result is a readiness to file an action to disavow paternity, with its implicit rejection of the child, and if need be to end the relationship altogether. Men who experience some trigger event will find a "cultural script" to guide response to their predicament that gives little or no place to empathy, care, and caution.

The powers of legislators and judges to heal fractured relationships are limited. In deciding a disestablishment case in December 2001, the justices of the Wyoming Supreme Court confronted the tragic dimension of their work: "Courts simply are not always capable of resolving the sorts of profound human dilemmas that are brought to their doorsteps, at least not in a way that will avoid all potential hardship to even innocent parties. Here, though Child has two presumptive fathers, he has none who wishes to fully embrace that role and the responsibility that goes with it" (*R.W.R. v. E.K.B.* 2001). Gearing the law toward modest goals of achieving greater consistency and minimizing harm, especially to innocent children, may be the best policy. In his special concurrence in the Wyoming case, Justice Michael Golden, joined by Chief Justice Larry Lehman, stated that while the "legal system certainly cannot bring love into a family," it should "at least provide a clear and coherent process when called upon to define a family." Adoption of this sober approach does not, of course, preclude hope that generosity and affection will triumph eventually. An Iowa man protested the continuation of a duty of support to a son with whom he had at one time enjoyed a warm, loving relationship, labeling it a "charade." The court rejected this characterization of the outcome of the disestablishment proceeding, expressing its hope that in the end the father's "heart will follow his money" (*Dye v. Geiger* 1996).

ACKNOWLEDGMENTS

This chapter draws on research funded by the National Institutes of Health, Grant No. R01 HG02485-01, "Genetic Ties and the Future of the Family." The views expressed are the author's own and do not represent the opinions or policies of the National

Institutes of Health. The author thanks Mark A. Rothstein for guidance and support and for suggesting the typology of responses. The research assistance of Elizabeth Stepien is also gratefully acknowledged. Some of the material in this chapter previously appeared in an article in the *Journal of the Center for Families, Children, and the Courts* 4 (2003): 3–26.

BIBLIOGRAPHY

Altenbernd, C. W. 1999. Quasi-marital children: The common law's failure in Privette and Daniel calls for statutory reform. *Florida State University Law Review* 26:219–83.

American Law Institute. 2002. *Principles of the Law of Family Dissolution: Analysis and Recommendations.* Newark, NJ: LexisNexis.

Anderlik, M. R. 2003. Disestablishment suits: What hath science wrought? *Journal of the Center for Families, Children, and the Courts* 4:3–26.

B.E.B. v. R.L.B. 1999. 979 P.2d 514 (Alaska).

Brady, M. 2001. DNA testing is causing state courts to relook at laws regarding paternity. *All Things Considered,* 9 April. Washington, DC: National Public Radio.

Brinkley v. King. 1997. 701 A.2d 176, 249 (Pa.).

Caron v. Caron. 1998. Ohio App. LEXIS 5653 (Ohio Ct. App.).

Caron v. Manfresca. 1999. Ohio App. LEXIS 4395 (Ohio Ct. App.).

The CBS Morning Show. 2000. 18 April. New York: CBS.

Citizens against Paternity Fraud. 2005. www.PaternityFraud.com.

Clevenger v. Clevenger. 1961. 189 Cal.App.2d 658 (Cal. Ct. App.).

Dads against Discrimination. 2002. www.dadsusa.com.

D.B.S. v. M.S. 1995. 888 P.2d 875 (Kan. Ct. App.), *aff'd* 903 P.2d 1345 (Kan. 1995).

Dye v. Geiger. 1996. 554 N.W.2d 538, 541 (Iowa).

Economist. 1999. Science and technology: Paternity test. 350:74.

Ex parte Jenkins. 1998. 723 So.2d 649, 678 (Ala.).

Follick, J. 2000. Court to rule on DNA impact on child support. *Tampa Tribune,* 20 August.

Gammon v. Cobb. 1976. 335 So.2d 261, 265 (Fla.).

Geen v. Geen. 1995. 666 So.2d 1192, 1197 (La. Ct. App.).

Glennon, T. 2000. Somebody's child: Evaluating the erosion of the marital presumption of paternity. *West Virginia Law Review* 102:547–605.

———. 2001. Expendable children: Defining belonging in a broken world. *Duke Journal of Gender Law and Policy* 8:269–83.

Goldstein, J., A. Freud, and A. J. Solnit. 1979. *Beyond the Best Interest of the Child.* New York: Free Press.

In re Caron. 2000. 744 N.E.2d 787 (Ohio Ct. Common Pleas).

In re Cheryl. 2001. 746 N.E.2d 488, 495 (Mass.).

In re Jacqueline S. 2001. Conn. Super. LEXIS 3570, 6 (Conn. Super. Ct.).

In re J.W.T. 1994. 872 S.W.2d 189, 197 (Tex.).

In re Marriage of A.J.N. & J.M.N. 1987. 414 N.W.2d 68 (Wis. Ct. App.).

Langston v. Riffe. 2000. 754 A.2d 389 (Md.).

Merkel v. Doe. 1993. 635 N.E.2d 70, 493 (Ohio Ct. Common Pleas).

Michael H. v. Gerald D. 1989. 491 U.S. 110, 118, 148.

Miscovich v. Miscovich. 1997. 688 A.2d 726 (Pa. Super. Ct. 1997), *aff'd,* 720 A.2d 764 (Pa. 1998), *cert. denied,* 526 U.S. 1113 (1999).

Murray, T. 1996. *The Worth of a Child.* Berkeley and Los Angeles: University of California Press.

N.A.H. v. S.L.S. 2000. 9 P.3d 354, 365 (Colo.).

Nelkin, D., and S. Lindee. 1995. *The DNA Mystique: The Gene as a Cultural Icon.* New York: W. H. Freeman.

Quinn, C. 2001. As DNA tests rule out paternity, men sue to stop support payments. *Atlanta Journal and Constitution,* 16 May.

Rubright v. Arnold. 1999. 973 P.2d 580 (Alaska).

R.W.R. v. E.K.B. 2001. 35 P.3d, 1224, 1228, 1232 (Wyo.).

Sants, H. J. 1964. Genealogical bewilderment in children with substitute parents. *British Journal of Medical Psychology* 37:133.

Smith v. Cole. 1989. 553 So.2d 847 (La.).

Smith v. Dep't of Human Resources. 1997. 487 S.E.2d 94, 96 (Ga. Ct. App.).

Stanley, A. 2002. So, who's your daddy? In DNA tests, TV finds elixir to raise ratings. *New York Times,* 19 March.

State v. Kovac. 1999. 984 P.2d 1109 (Alaska).

Strauser v. Stahr. 1999. 726 A.2d 176 (Pa.).

Tandra S. v. Tyrone W. 1994. 648 A.2d 439 (Md.).

Wise v. Fryar. 2001. 49 S.W.3d 450 (Tex. Ct. App.).

CHAPTER ELEVEN

Assisted Reproductive Technology and the Challenge for Paternity Laws

Lori B. Andrews, J.D.

Since the dawn of humankind, adults have had to assume responsibility for the care of children. The means of assigning that responsibility through the ages have reflected the cultural values of any given generation. Thus, evolving concepts—such as illegitimacy, children as chattel, the tender years doctrine, the psychological parent, joint custody, preconception intent, and the presumption of a husband's parentage of children of the marriage—all reflect the cultural mores of their times and further particular societal goals. The goals may vary widely by generation, from underscoring male dominance to discouraging adultery, from rewarding loving bonds to protecting the state's treasury, from punishing homosexual parenthood to facilitating it. In this chapter I analyze the cultural values at play in attempts to assign parental rights and responsibilities on the basis of genetics, including parental rights and responsibilities for children conceived through assisted reproductive technology.

It is a paradoxical time for examining the role of genetics in the assignment of legal parenthood. In Chicago, where I live, divorced men take their children to Lincoln Park to play, then they pop into a nearby hospital for DNA testing to determine whether the child is really "theirs." If DNA testing excludes them as genetic dads, some take to the courts to attempt to avoid paying child support. In some cases, on advice of counsel, they stop seeing the child they had parented for years in order to "strengthen their case."

At that same hospital, other men—those with infertility problems—join their wives to use donated semen to create a child of the marriage. These men consider themselves the father of the resulting child, despite their lack of a genetic connection to the child.

The evolving court cases on reproductive technologies and on DNA paternity testing raise fascinating questions about the role of the public and private realms in establishing parental rights and obligations. Legal parenthood has generally been defined by statutes and case law. A recurrent theme is that parental rights and responsibilities may not be assigned by private contract. Yet, in the realm of reproductive technologies, contract-like principles are increasingly being used to determine who are mommy and daddy. At the same time, public institutions such as courts do not have a monopoly on ordering DNA testing to determine parenthood. With the proliferation of private companies touting their DNA testing services via billboards and Web sites, putative and presumed fathers are seeking private tests on themselves and their children.

Determination of legal parenthood previously focused primarily on the trinity of mother, father, and child, but now an assortment of other individuals are in the legal spotlight as well. With reproductive technologies, a child might have five or more parents—such as the sperm provider, egg provider, woman who carries the child, and the couple who intend to raise the child. And when a child has been conceived through sexual intercourse, but the father subsequently dies, courts have had to adjudicate the question of whether the putative father's relatives may be subjected to DNA testing to determine whether a particular child should share in the decedent's estate.

The Role of Biology and Social Criteria in Parenthood Determinations

The legal assignment of parental rights and responsibilities over children has combined both biological and social criteria. For countless generations, maternal rights over children were easy to assign. The woman who gave birth to the child was the legal mother. This concept still prevails in the language of the parentage laws of many states. For example, California has a statutory provision that a parent-child relationship may be established "between a child and the natural mother . . . by proof of her having given birth to the child" (Cal. Family Code § 7610).

With respect to fathers, determination of legal parenthood has been more complicated. In large measure, paternity has been based on social, rather than biological, factors. Paternity statutes generally provide that, if a woman is married, her husband is the father of her child, unless the husband proves he was sterile or had no access to the wife at the time of conception (e.g., he was away at sea for months). If the woman was not married and either she or the state wanted to assert that a man was the legal father, legal fatherhood was assigned based on the man's biological connection to the child. However, in situations in which the child had passed infancy and the unwed mother wanted to give the child to a stranger for adoption or have the child adopted by her subsequent spouse, and the biological father objected, a mere biological bond was insufficient for the man to establish paternity. Generally, when an unmarried biological father is trying to gain rights to a child, he must show that he has some social relation with that child. In *Lehr v. Robertson* (1983), for example, an unmarried father petitioned to vacate the order of adoption of his two-year-old child by the mother's husband. The biological father, however, had never supported the child or entered his name into a putative father registry. The U.S. Supreme Court held that the biological father's due process and equal protection rights were not violated by his failing to receive notice and an opportunity to be heard before his child was adopted, because the father had never had any significant custodial, personal, or financial relationship with the child. This "social" approach to legal fatherhood serves important goals, such as protecting marriages and assuring support for children. Thus courts have considered it to be in the best interests of the child for the husband of the woman who gave birth to be declared the legal father.

Now, though, the social test for fatherhood is increasingly being replaced by a genetic one. DNA paternity tests can demonstrate to a high degree of certainty (99% or higher) who the biological father is, thereby generating questions about whether a biological assignment of fatherhood should replace the social one within marriage. Should the husband be able to authorize DNA testing on the child without the mother's consent to determine whether he is the biological father? Should such DNA testing be done only on the basis of a court order? If the couple divorces, should the ex-husband be able to sever ties with a child he reared for years, simply on the grounds that he was not the sperm provider? What about the ex-husband who wants custody of a child with whom he has a loving bond, but who is told by the ex-wife that he should have no rights because he is not actually the child's biological father? Courts are currently struggling with the question of whether a genetic test indicating a high probability of paternity should trump other means of establishing legal fatherhood. Questions have arisen about whether genetic paternity testing, with its high level of accuracy, should displace the social relationship model when sexual reproduction creates a child—and whether that same testing should be completely irrelevant when reproductive technologies are used. Yet in both instances, the decision about genetic testing should be made with concern for the social values—such as concerns about the stability of family structures and the emotional and financial well-being of children—that the previous legal scheme attempted to embody. Any new legal scheme should also demonstrate adequate concern about the ethical and cultural issues raised by genetic testing itself.

DNA Testing in the Context of Sexual Reproduction

The high level of accuracy with which DNA testing correlates with genetic parenthood is fostering widespread adoption of such testing to determine legal parenthood, with little regard for other social values at stake. Yet such testing raises important questions of authorization and closure. It touches on values such as ensuring the psychological and financial well-being of children and the privacy of relatives.

Issues arise at various points in the process of paternity determination. There are dilemmas about who should be able to authorize DNA paternity testing and under what circumstances. There are questions about whether such information should be admissible in court and, if so, what impact it should have. There are also issues of closure. Should the parties be able to relitigate issues of parenthood each time a newer, more accurate paternity test is developed? Should a lover be able to require DNA testing of the child of a married couple over the couple's objection? Should a divorced man be able to relitigate questions of child support after private paternity testing and, if so, under what circumstances? There are also questions about how far society should go in attempting to establish legal paternity when the putative father is missing or dead. Should blood relatives be forced to be tested? Should a putative father's corpse be exhumed and tested?

Currently, all these questions are being addressed in a hodge-podge of ways by courts, legislators, and the proponents of model laws. Often, the positions taken by these disparate decision makers clash or show little regard for the personal and social values at stake. My own opinion is that young children's financial support and emotional well-being should be primary concerns in policy development, but that concerns about privacy should also have a role.

Authorization of Paternity Testing

There is very little legal authority regarding who may authorize DNA paternity tests and whether such testing should ever be done surreptitiously. Should an individual be able to use saliva from a glass, a hair follicle from a comb, or tissue from discarded dental floss to test someone's DNA without his knowledge or consent? The 2000 iteration of the Uniform Parentage Act (UPA), adopted by the National Conference of Commissioners on Uniform State Laws, does not address how DNA samples are collected (when testing is performed outside a court proceeding). And testing laboratories, especially those with home testing services, often do not inquire into the source of the sample.

The very nature of private paternity testing needs to be assessed. A strong policy argument could be made that it is not in the best interests of children to allow presumed fathers to surreptitiously test children without maternal consent, except in the context of a judicial proceeding such as a divorce. In fact, I would favor an approach that does not allow paternity testing outside the legal system. In Nevada, paternity testing without informed consent may be done only under a court order (Nev. Rev. Stat. 629.151). In Vermont, the law says that "no person shall be required to undergo genetic testing" (Vt. Stat. Title 18 § 9332[a]) and allows parentage testing only if "required by law" (Vt. Stat. Title 18 § 9332[b]).

Even when courts themselves order DNA testing, they might be doing so in inappropriate circumstances. For example, if a genetic test will be completely irrelevant to the court's determination of legal parenthood, it would seem inappropriate for the court to order such testing. In the case of *N.A.H. v. S.L.S.* (2000), a married woman's lover brought suit to establish his paternity of her one-and-a-half-year-old child, for whom he had been caring ten hours a week. A magistrate ordered DNA testing and, based on the result, declared the lover the biological and legal father. The magistrate ordered that the child's name be changed and that the parties work with a psychologist to integrate the biological father into the child's life. On appeal, the Colorado Supreme Court noted that both DNA testing and marriage to the woman created rebuttable presumptions of paternity. The court said DNA testing is the most accurate way to determine paternity "unless this presumption is outweighed by consideration of public policy." The court reversed the magistrate's order to declare the biological father to be the legal father. Instead, the court held parenthood should be determined by the "best interests of the child versus biology." Unfortunately, the married couple was unsuccessful in arguing that the best interests standards should be applied earlier—before a decision to order paternity testing is made by the court. Yet DNA paternity testing without legal effect can be unnecessarily disruptive.

Closure

Courts and legislatures that favor DNA paternity testing to establish legal fatherhood are struggling with the question of whether there should be a limited time period during which the test result may be used. The concern is obviously for the psychological well-being of the child; once he or she is past a certain age, adding or subtracting a father in the family may be disruptive.

Closure is an issue in attempts both to include and to exclude men as fathers. In some cases, it may be the mother who wishes to introduce genetic evidence to prove paternity of an older child. *S.C.G. v. J.G.Y.* (2000) raised the issue of whether paternity should be relitigated each time an improved test becomes available. The biological mother of the child filed a paternity action against two men she thought could be the father of her child. The results of human leukocyte antigen testing (a 95% accurate test that examines proteins on the surface of white blood cells) excluded both men from being the father of the child. Seven years later, one of the previously excluded men underwent DNA testing, which established a 99.9 percent probability of paternity. When the mother requested the paternity case be reopened based on that evidence, the court was not willing to do so. The court held that reopening the paternity action would not be in the best interests of the child.

Likewise, it seems inappropriate to allow divorced fathers or former lovers to use DNA testing indefinitely to reopen child support responsibilities. In another case, the child was nine years old at the time of the legal action (*Tyrone W. v. Danielle R.* 1999). Given that social values regarding the best interests of the child rather than biological ties are the basis of the legal rule that a child born to a married woman is her husband's child, DNA paternity testing should not be used to disrupt that equation, particularly if the husband has developed a bond with the child. In one case, a seven-year-old boy was diagnosed with cystic fibrosis, a recessive disorder in which both parents must be carriers to have an affected child. Because he was not a carrier of the cystic fibrosis mutation, the boy's "father" realized that his "son" was not his biological child. However, the court did not let him reopen the final divorce decree confirming fatherhood, because the man knew his wife had been unfaithful and yet he had not sought paternity testing at the time of the divorce (*Wise v. Fryar* 2001). In another case, the Pennsylvania Supreme Court refused to let an ex-husband use DNA paternity tests to stop paying child support, because he had not established by clear and convincing evidence nonaccess, sterility, or impotency under the state statute (*Miscovich v. Miscovich* 1997). The court ruled that allowing the ex-husband to rebut paternity after the divorce could threaten family interests. Now some attorneys advise all men to request paternity testing at the time of divorce.

Some courts have been unwilling to reopen paternity cases based on DNA tests, but a few legislatures have begun to pass laws allowing such an action, often in response to particular court cases holding a nonbiological dad responsible for child support. In Maryland, Tyrone W. acknowledged paternity of Tandra S.'s child, which was incorporated into a court judgment. He agreed to pay child support and she agreed to allow visitation. When the child was two, Tyrone filed to set aside the judgment on the basis of "fraud," because blood tests excluded him as a father. An appellate court ruled that the concept of fraud to support reopening of a judgment did not cover facts intrinsic to the case itself (*Tandra S. v. Tyrone W.* 1994). The court held that Tyrone W. must continue paying child support.

In his dissenting opinion, one of the justices in the case ignored the social values at stake in a paternity action:

> In a paternity action, unlike other lawsuits, a court is called upon to declare a scientific, biological fact, namely whether a particular individual is the biological father of a given child . . . Under the majority's view, presumably if the Provincial Court of Maryland in the 1600's had issued a decree that the earth was flat, the absence of 'fraud, mistake or irregularity,' as narrowly defined by this Court, would make that Provincial Court decree sacrosanct. Or if Rule 2-535(b) were to be given extra-territorial effect, presumably the March 5, 1616, decree by a tribunal in Rome, aimed at Galileo Galilei, and declaring that Copernicanism is erroneous and that the planet earth is the center of the universe, would be given conclusive effect.

Apparently, Maryland legislators were convinced by the logic of the dissent. The following year, they passed a statute providing that a paternity order may be set aside if a blood test or genetic test excludes the individual as the father (Md. Code Ann. Fam. Law § 5-1038). Tyrone W. went back to court—this time to challenge his status as the legal father of a child born to a different woman

(*Tyrone W. v. Danielle R.* 1999). Even though the child was nine years old at the time and Tyrone W.'s paternity had been acknowledged before the passage of the statute, the court held it could be applied retroactively to allow a challenge to paternity based on the genetic test.

The Maryland statute, which is being copied in other states, allows a genetic test to upset paternity judgments at any time in the child's life. This may be in the putative father's best interests, but it is not in the child's best interests. Bills have been proposed to allow a man to stop paying child support and recover previously paid support if DNA paternity testing shows he is not the father. Such actions could thrust the woman (and child) into poverty.

At the very least, there should be time limitations on paternity testing. The UPA (§ 607[a]) gives presumed fathers two years after the child's birth to contest paternity. That seems to be a reasonable amount of time to give suspicious husbands a chance to dispute paternity and yet protect children over age two who develop relationships with presumed fathers.

There are also closure issues when a putative father dies. Postmortem paternity testing has been authorized on frozen blood samples. In other instances, corpses have been disinterred for paternity testing. Some states set time bars on paternity actions by children. In *Rushford v. Caines* (2001), a woman in her forties learned through an anonymous note that a man who died testate (i.e., with a will) might be her biological father. She brought an action in probate court to release the decedent's DNA for testing, but the court applied a provision of the Ohio paternity statute that bars an action brought by a child more than five years after the child reaches age eighteen. The court was unpersuaded by her argument that the statute of limitations should have been tolled during the period she did not know the decedent might be her biological father.

When a putative father has died, it may be appropriate to allow testing on existing tissue samples—or, in rare cases, to disinter the body. The UPA (§ 509) allows disinterment "for good cause shown." However, time limits should be put on disinterment, depending on the age of the child. One approach would be to prohibit disinterment after the child reaches age eighteen. The policy goal of providing support for the rearing of the child has already been missed, so there is less need for such an action if paternity has not been acknowledged during the child's minority. Moreover, disinterment should not be ordered unless there is strong evidence of a relationship between the deceased and the mother.

Testing the Putative Father's Other Children and Relatives

In other realms, both law and medicine increasingly tread carefully before DNA testing is undertaken. In 1993, the federal Office for Protection from Research Risks (now known as the Office for Human Research Protections) indicated that DNA testing should be considered as raising "more than minimal risks." Obtaining blood from a person for identification in the criminal context is considered a search and seizure under the Fourth Amendment (*Jones v. Murray* 1992). Medical interventions without consent violate an individual's constitutional right to liberty (when undertaken by a state actor or under color of state law) (*Cruzan v. Director, Missouri Department of Health* 1990) and common law right of bodily integrity (*Union Pac. Ry. Co. v. Botsford* 1891).

The reason for ordering paternity testing on a putative father is to identify him to require him to meet his parental responsibilities. Perhaps because courts have not had to engage in lengthy analysis to facilitate such an approach, they have thoughtlessly slipped into ordering DNA testing on relatives of deceased putative fathers without sufficient analysis.

In *Lach v. Welch* (1997), Michael Welch had a child with his wife. He also had a lover, Sharon Lach, who had a three-year-old daughter, Kaitlin. After Michael's death in an auto accident, Sharon sought to establish that Michael was Kaitlin's father. She asked the court to order paternity testing on Michael's mother and on the minor child of Michael's marriage. The court, operating on the assumption that testing the paternal grandparents would be of higher accuracy than testing the decedent's remains, mandated the testing.

Similarly, in *Sudwischer v. Estate of Hoffpauir* (1991), the Supreme Court of Louisiana affirmed an order that Rosemary, the legitimate daughter of a deceased father, provide a blood test to determine whether another woman, Alana, was the deceased man's illegitimate daughter. The court determined that Alana had a constitutional right to prove filiation, an "overriding emotional and financial interest in knowing her father's identity."

Other courts have considered it appropriate to order testing of the mother of a decedent's other children, even if she will not inherit under the will. A New Jersey court held, for example, that "a court has inherent power to order anyone within its jurisdiction to submit to such tests when they are needed to adjudicate a genuine issue before it" (*In re Estate of Rogers* 1990). Even though the court indicated that DNA paternity testing implicated

Fourth Amendment concerns, the court held that the ex-wife could be held in contempt of court for refusing testing. The appellate court did not go as far as the lower court, which suggested that the ex-wife's refusal to undergo testing was *proof* of the husband's paternity of another woman's child. The decision is particularly disturbing because the test was ordered on very little proof that the husband fathered the illegitimate child. The evidence consisted of the following: "The decedent's military records corroborated plaintiff's mother's testimony that he was in the vicinity of where she lived when plaintiffs were conceived."

Other judges have criticized the idea of testing relatives other than the putative dad. Such judges express concerns about the social values at stake beyond the financial support of the child. They raise issues about the privacy interests of the relatives and express concerns about the actions of a governmental institution (the court) forcing DNA testing on an individual who has no duty to support the child.

The dissenting judge in *Sudwischer,* for example, criticized the majority for not focusing on the most important constitutional rights at issue—Rosemary's federal and state constitutional rights to be free from unreasonable invasions or intrusions of her body. The dissent cited U.S. Supreme Court cases, including *Cruzan v. Director, Missouri Department of Health* (1990), *Griswold v. Connecticut* (1965), and *Whalen v. Roe* (1977), to underscore how repugnant any invasion of bodily integrity is to the values of liberty, physical freedom, self-determination, and the ability to make important decisions. The dissent in *Sudwischer* stated further that, although Alana did not demonstrate any affirmative act of the state to deny her rights, Rosemary could show state action in the form of an order requiring her to submit to genetic testing. Because only a narrowly drawn means to further a compelling state interest would outweigh Rosemary's constitutional rights, the dissenting judge would not have ordered the test. The dissenting judge noted that the state's interests were "limited and even minimal." Because siblings and other collateral relatives do not have a duty to support a child, there is no justification for requiring them to undergo genetic testing.

The situation could be analogized to cases in which judges have recognized a right to refuse blood testing to aid family members in need of transplants. In *Curran v. Bosze* (1990), the Illinois Supreme Court denied the request of a father to submit his three-and-a-half-year-old twins to blood tests (over the objection of their mother, the custodial parent) to determine their compatibility as bone marrow donors for their half brother.

Privacy-based arguments do occasionally prevail in paternity cases. In *William M. v. Superior Court* (1990), a California appellate court held that the paternity statute did not authorize the court to mandate DNA testing of the deceased man's parents. The attorney for the child had made the clever argument that, because the grandparents could themselves bring an action to establish paternity in order to gain visitation rights, the child had an equal protection claim to DNA testing of the grandparents. The court rejected the argument due to concerns about invading the grandparents' privacy. The court was also concerned about the range of relatives who might be called in if DNA paternity testing beyond the mother, father, and child were allowed. "If Michael [the putative father] had no living parents, we might well be addressing identical issues involving Michael's brothers and sisters, cousins or other relatives. Given these troubling implications the decision of who may properly be made a party defendant in a paternity action subject to mandatory blood testing is one for the Legislature."

In *Estate of Sanders* (1992), in an action by the decedent's alleged child conceived with a lover, the court refused to mandate DNA testing of the mothers of the decedent's acknowledged adult children. The court was concerned about the privacy invasion. The court also reasoned that the other mothers could not be brought in as parties, because they had no financial interest in the decedent's estate. The judge ruled that DNA testing should be done only if there was evidence of paternity while the man was alive, such as a paternity action or the man's activities in holding out the child as his own.

The UPA (§ 508) authorizes the genetic testing of a man's parents, his siblings, his other children, or his other relatives if genetic samples are "not available" from the man who may be the father of the child. Such a provision—as well as cases that take a similar tack—do not give sufficient consideration to the privacy interests and convenience of relatives. What if the putative father lives in another state or is away at war? Why should his relatives be hauled into court for genetic testing? Even if such a provision were interpreted just to cover situations in which the man was dead, the provision is not justified. These relatives are under no obligation to support the child, whatever the result of testing, so they seem an inappropriate subject of such a court-ordered intervention. In addition, particularly with respect to young legitimate children of the deceased man, the procedure may be emotionally detrimental. The testing of relatives also sends an inappropriate policy message—that mandatory genetic testing can be undertaken on individuals who have not engaged in any behavior

that could lead to legal responsibility. The UPA shows no sensitivity to these issues. It erroneously assumes that the lack of physical intrusiveness of the genetic test means that it has little or no social or personal impact. For example,
the comment to § 508 of the UPA 2000 dealing with testing relatives states,
"Genetic testing in the modern age is not invasive—use of the buccal swab
method means that the intrusion into the privacy of the individual is relatively
slight compared to the right of the child to have parentage established."

The UPA of 2000 does contain some limiting language on the testing of relatives. Section 508(b) states that such testing should be done only if the "need
for genetic testing outweighs the legitimate interests of the individual sought
to be tested." In my own analysis, the legitimate right of relatives to refuse
genetic testing would be considered of such importance that testing would
never be undertaken in the face of such a refusal.

Parentage and Assisted Reproductive Technologies

Although genetic testing is becoming more commonplace as a means to assign legal parenthood of children conceived through sexual intercourse, it is
increasingly irrelevant with most new reproductive technologies. Such technologies are challenging the traditional determination of maternity and paternity. An infertile woman can contract with an egg donor and a surrogate
mother to bear a child for her. Which of these three mothers—genetic, gestational, or social—should be considered the legal mother? Who is the legal father when donor sperm is used? In such cases, assignment of legal parenthood
relies less on biology and more on social constructs, looking at the intent of
the parties before conception to determine who should bear rights and responsibilities with respect to the child. Even when genetic testing plays a role
in the determination of legal fatherhood in the context of reproductive technologies—as it does when posthumous conception occurs—the man's intent
to father a child after his death also must be proven.

Artificial Insemination by Donor

Generally, state statutes provide that the husband of a woman who con-
ceives during marriage or within a certain number of days thereafter is presumed to be the father of the child and has legal responsibilities for his or her
rearing. Some of these statutes, however, present problems with respect to reproductive technologies. Some provide an exception to the presumption of

paternity if the husband is sterile. Thus a husband who is sterile but who wants to be considered the legal father of a child born to his wife after donor insemination may not be adequately protected. In cases of divorce, some women have tried to deny their ex-husband visitation rights to the child created by donor insemination, on the grounds that he was not the biological father, and some men have tried to stop supporting the child on the same grounds. In some cases, the divorce dispute is the first time the child learns that his social dad is not his biological dad.

To avoid financial and psychological harm to the child, at least thirty-four states have adopted laws providing that the resulting child is the legal offspring of the sperm recipient and her consenting husband. Even in the absence of a statute on artificial insemination, courts today are likely to hold that a consenting husband is the legal father of the resulting child. In a California case, *People v. Sorensen* (1968), the court held that an infertile man who consents to his wife's artificial insemination using a third-party donor cannot disclaim responsibility after the child is born. The court in the *Sorensen* case also pointed out that it would be unreasonable to ask the donor to support the child: "The anonymous donor of the sperm cannot be considered the 'natural father,' as he is no more responsible for the use made of his sperm than is the donor of blood or a kidney."

Most of the state statutes governing artificial insemination specifically refer to the insemination of a *wife* and make her husband the legal father. Questions of paternity arise in these states when an unmarried woman is artificially inseminated. A single woman's intent to parent without input from the sperm donor may be compromised by statutory provisions that cover only married women or apply only to situations in which a physician is involved in the procedure. Doctors are not necessary to the process (a woman can inseminate herself using a turkey baster), but at least sixteen of the related statutes assume that artificial insemination by donor (AID) will be performed by or under the supervision of a "licensed physician," "certified medical doctor," or person "duly authorized to practice medicine." Because AID is a relatively simple procedure and involves minimal risks, the statutes that require medical assistance raise questions about whether its performance by someone other than a physician (such as a husband, lover, donor, or friend) should have legal consequences for determining parentage.

The statutory requirement for physician supervision creates problems when AID performed by a nonphysician involves an unmarried woman. Some unmarried women have trouble finding physicians who will agree to perform the procedure for them. Their alternative is to find a donor through a network of friends and acquaintances. In California, an unmarried woman privately selected a sperm donor and performed the insemination herself in her home (*Jhordan C. v. Mary K.* 1986). The sperm donor was listed as the father on the child's birth certificate. He filed an action to establish paternity and visitation rights. The appellate court scrutinized the statute, which said, "The donor of semen provided to a licensed physician for use in artificial insemination of a woman other than the donor's wife is treated in law as if he were not the natural father of a child thereby conceived" (Cal. Civ. Code § 7005[b]). The court held that, because the semen was not provided to a physician, the donor was the legal father, and it granted him visitation rights. Yet it seems implausible that the legislature actually intended the determination of paternity to hinge on whether a doctor was involved in the process.

Indeed, the court noted that "nothing inherent in artificial insemination requires the involvement of a physician" (*Jhordan C. v. Mary K.* 1986). Physician involvement "might offend a woman's sense of privacy and reproductive autonomy, might result in burdensome costs to some women, and might interfere with a woman's desire to conduct the procedure in a comfortable environment such as her own home or to choose the donor herself." A third reason for not using the services of a physician, not mentioned by the court, is that some people feel that the medical screening of donors by infertility clinics is inadequate and thus they wish to choose their own donors. The court also gave two reasons why physician involvement might be appropriate, however. The physician could obtain a medical history of the donor and screen him. Also, the physician "can serve to create a formal, documented structure for the donor-recipient relationship to avoid misunderstandings between the parties."

Because of the difficulty some unmarried women have had in using artificial insemination to create a child without a legal father, the AID statutes in some states (such as Ohio and Oregon) try to clarify this issue by providing that, if an unmarried woman is artificially inseminated, "the donor shall not be treated in law or regarded as the natural father." In *McIntyre v. Crouch* (1989), the donor and mother were acquainted but unmarried. In that case, the donor/father gave his semen to the mother, but later brought a filiation action against her, claiming that he had acted in reliance on an agreement with the mother that he would remain active in the child's life and enjoy visitation rights. The mother denied the agreement, and the court refused to distinguish the father from an anonymous donor for purposes of the Oregon statute barring him from asserting parental rights. While rejecting the father's state constitutional claims, the court conceded that, if the father could prove the existence of the alleged agreement regarding his parental rights, the Oregon statute as applied to him would violate his federal Fourteenth Amendment due process rights. The court decreed that "a state may not place an absolute bar to a biological father's efforts to assert the rights and responsibilities of fatherhood" (*McIntyre v. Crouch* 1989; *Lehr v. Robertson* 1983). A concurring judge asserted that the legislative history of the Oregon statute barring parental rights of sperm donors revealed that it was not intended to apply to these unique circumstances.

In another Oregon case, *Leckie v. Voorhies* (1994), a known sperm donor who signed an explicit waiver to any rights of guardianship or custody filed a petition to establish paternity and visitation. He claimed that the conduct of the parties implicitly modified their agreement. The mother and her female partner had moved into a house owned by the donor on land next door to his home, he visited the child several hours per week, and he made substantial financial contributions for the child's benefit. The appellate court, however, found that unlike the situation in *McIntyre,* here the agreement expressly and effectively waived any entitlement the sperm donor may have had to parental rights, including any assertion of filiation.

Egg Donation

Historically, there was no need for "maternity statutes" to indicate who the mother was. The woman who gave birth was invariably both the genetic and gestational mother. Her delivery of the child was enough for the law to assign her legal motherhood. But as motherhood has become more radically separated into its constituent parts—genetic, gestational, and social—new statutes are necessary to clarify who has what rights.

Currently, only five states have laws specifically addressing parentage in egg donation. Each of these statutes irrebuttably presumes that a child resulting from egg donation is the child of the couple who consented to receive the donated egg. The egg recipient in many other states would have a strong claim to the resulting child. Because traditional law recognized the woman who gives birth as the legal mother, so the woman who gestates an embryo created with a donor egg will be presumed to be the mother. In states without an egg donation statute, there is nonetheless a small chance that the donor of an unfertilized or fertilized egg would be able to sue to claim parental rights to the resulting child. Numerous *paternity* acts (originally enacted to assign legal fatherhood) describe in broad language the person who may bring an action to claim legal parenthood. A genetic, but not gestating, mother (the egg donor) would seem to fall within the categories of mother, interested party, or relative who may bring actions under the various state paternity acts. In addition, even in states where statutes do not explicitly allow women to claim legal parenthood of a child born to another woman, the egg donor might be able to raise a constitutional equal protection claim. Many state paternity acts have provisions that allow a biological father to claim parenthood of a child born to someone other than his wife. Conceivably, a court could hold that it would violate equal protection principles to deny a woman the right to bring an action under the paternity statutes to establish her legal parenthood to a child born to someone else, such as in an action by an egg donor to assert rights of visitation or custody to the child created with her egg.

Surrogate Motherhood

In traditional surrogacy, the surrogate mother is artificially inseminated with the sperm of the husband of an infertile woman. Thus the traditional surrogate provides an egg and gestates the fetus. In many states, this creates the possibility of conflicts about legal parenthood if the surrogate mother changes her mind and wants to keep the child. Under existing legal principles, the surrogate mother has a strong claim to be recognized as the legal mother. Moreover, her husband could readily be seen as the legal father. Since this is not the result the parties initially intended, various surrogacy cases have entered the courts.

In one Michigan case, a man whose sperm had been used to inseminate a surrogate filed suit under the Paternity Act for a declaration of his paternity, but the trial court and the appellate court held that the statute could not be used to determine the paternity of a child born to a surrogate (*Syrkowski v. Appleyard* 1983). The Michigan Supreme Court reversed, holding that the state's Paternity Act does allow a father to establish paternity, even if the drafters of the act had not specifically envisioned the surrogate mother situation (*Syrkowski v. Appleyard* 1985). However, a subsequently enacted Michigan statute provides that "a surrogate parentage contract is void and unenforceable as contrary to public policy" (Michigan Comp. Laws Ann. § 722.855 2002). In fact, the Michigan law so frowns upon surrogacy that it provides criminal penalties. With respect to surrogate parentage contracts in general (where there is no issue of a party without legal capacity), the Michigan criminal law provides that a person shall not "enter into, induce, arrange, procure, or otherwise assist in the formation of a surrogate parentage contract for compensation" (Mich. Comp. Laws Ann. § 722.857[1] 2002).

Beyond the issue of whether the man providing the sperm will be recognized as the legal father, questions arise as to whether a surrogate who provides an egg and gestates a fetus should be able to change her mind and gain custody of the child. In *In re Baby M.* (1988a), the New Jersey Supreme Court held that the adoption laws should apply to traditional surrogacy. Those laws allow a biological mother a certain time period after birth to decide to retain custody of the child. Consequently, the *Baby M.* court recognized the surrogate as the legal mother and the man providing the sperm as the legal father. The New Jersey Supreme Court awarded continuing physical custody to the intended father and his wife in *In re Baby M.* (1988a), but remanded to the lower court the issue of visitation rights for Mary Beth Whitehead-Gould, the surrogate mother. Ultimately the court awarded Whitehead two days' weekly visitation, certain holidays, and a two-week vacation each year (*In re Baby M.* 1988b).

A similar case arose in California. In *In re Moschetta* (1994), the surrogate was artificially inseminated with the sperm of the intended father. When he and his wife subsequently had marital problems, the pregnant surrogate said she would turn the baby over to them only if they got marriage counseling. They did so for a while, but soon after the child's birth, the husband left the wife, taking the baby with him. When the couple separated, the surrogate sought custody. A California Superior Court Judge held that the surrogate had parental rights and that the intended mother had no parental rights because she had no biological relationship to the child. The court ignored the fact that the intended mother had raised the child for the child's first seven months. The court ruled that the surrogate and the intended father would co-parent the child; the child would live with the surrogate on weekdays during the day and with the intended father in the evenings and on weekends. An appellate court affirmed the findings that the husband and surrogate were the legal parents, but remanded as to the custody decision.

A surrogate will ordinarily not be allowed to change her mind after the statutory time period under the adoption act has passed, however. In *Adoption of Matthew B.* (1991), the surrogate agreed to an adoption by the intended parents, but later changed her mind and asked for custody of the eight-month-old child. The court ruled in favor of the intended parents, finding that their continued custody would be in the child's best interests.

About half the states have adopted statutes regulating surrogate parenting, but states vary in whether they address issues of legal parenthood—and, if so, how they address them. Some states use their paternity laws to attempt to discourage surrogate motherhood by providing that the surrogate and her husband are the legal parents, or that they are the legal parents unless the child is the genetic offspring of the contracting couple. In most cases, however, neither the intended parents nor the surrogate and her husband desire that outcome. Surrogates do not enter into these arrangements to make a baby for their own families.

Other states, such as Michigan and Washington, decide issues of custody based on an evaluation of each individual case and a determination of what is in the best interests of the child. However, is it really in the best interests of the child to leave custody open to challenge in every case? Might it not be better to assure that the child has a secure and definite home to go to? It would seem preferable to use the approach of those states that presume that the contracting couple/intended parents are the legal parents.

Surrogate Gestational Motherhood

The possibility of transferring a couple's embryo into a surrogate mother for gestation has added a new wrinkle to the litigation about surrogate motherhood. Since the gestational mother is generally considered to be the legal mother, it is likely that, in at least some jurisdictions, judges will hold that the surrogate gestational mother is the legal mother and will require the intended parents, or at least the intended mother, to adopt the child. But the surrogate gestational mother's claim will generally be weaker than if she had provided the egg as well.

When a surrogate gestational mother changes her mind and decides to assert parental rights to the child, she has an even more difficult time than a surrogate mother in obtaining custody of the child. In *Johnson v. Calvert* (1993), the California Supreme Court held that the genetic parents, not the surrogate gestational mother, were the legal parents of the resulting child and that such a result was not offensive to the state or federal constitution or to public policy. Applying the Uniform Parentage Act of 1973, the court concluded that both the genetic mother and the gestational mother had statutory claims to being the child's legal mother, because the act of 1973 allowed a woman to establish legal motherhood both through evidence of having given birth to the child and through genetic marker evidence derived from blood testing. Because there was undisputed evidence that the surrogate had given birth to the child, as well as undisputed evidence that the wife was genetically related to the child, both women produced evidence of a mother and child relationship as contemplated by the Uniform Parentage Act of 1973.

The court was then faced with the fact that California law recognizes only one legal mother for any child, despite advances in reproductive technology that render a different outcome biologically possible. Finding no clear legislative preference in the act of 1973 between blood testing evidence and proof of having given birth, the court concluded that an inquiry into the intent of the parties as manifested in the surrogacy agreement was required: "Although the Act recognizes both genetic consanguinity and giving birth as means of establishing a mother and child relationship, when the two means do not coincide in one woman, she who intended to procreate the child—that is, she who intended to bring about the birth of a child that she intended to raise as her own—is the natural mother under California law."

The court in *Johnson* next addressed the constitutionality of the determination that the surrogate gestational mother was not the legal mother. The court concluded that the surrogate's federal substantive due process, privacy, and procreative freedom claims all depended on a prior determination that she was indeed the resulting child's mother, which under California law she was not.

Moreover, the court found that even under the broader protections of the California Constitution, the surrogate's right of privacy was not violated. The court reasoned that the choice to gestate and deliver a baby to its genetic parents pursuant to a surrogacy agreement was not the constitutional equivalent of the decision to bear a child of one's own. The court explained, "A woman who enters into a gestational surrogacy arrangement is not exercising her own right to make procreative choices; she is agreeing to provide a necessary and profoundly important service without (by definition) any expectation that she will raise the resulting child as her own."

In re Marriage of Buzzanca (1998) raised new questions about surrogate parenting when the trial court held that the child, Jaycee, had no legal parents. The case differed from previous cases because it involved a surrogacy contract between four people—a husband and wife and the surrogate and her husband— whereby the surrogate was implanted with an embryo created by anonymous donors. After implantation of the embryo but before the birth of the child, the intended parents separated. Several months later, the wife brought an action for temporary child support for care of the child. The intended father claimed that under the Uniform Parentage Act of 1973, the surrogate mother was the lawful mother of the child because she gave birth to the child. The California Court of Appeal reversed the trial court's conclusion that Jaycee had no lawful parents and held that "even though neither Luanne nor John are biologically related to Jaycee, they are still her lawful parents given their initiating role as the intended parents in her conception and birth." The court held that the intended mother, Luanne, could be awarded custody of the child and that the intended father, John, could be held financially responsible for care of the child.

Posthumous Reproduction

Posthumous births, when a woman's husband or partner dies before their child's birth, have occurred throughout human history, but only recently has it become possible to create children with sperm from a man who has already died or is in a coma. Posthumous procreation is also possible through the use of frozen embryos and a surrogate (Sutton 1999).

Since the advent of cryopreservation, men have chosen to store their sperm for a variety of reasons. A common situation occurs when a man deposits his sperm in a sperm or tissue bank before undergoing a medical procedure that could result in sterility. Other men store sperm before entering active military service. In 2003, some sperm banks offered discounts to U.S. soldiers who wanted to store sperm before going to war against Iraq (Newbart 2003; Clark 2003).

Case law indicates that men should be able to arrange to create children after they die. It is unclear, though, whether their offspring will necessarily be recognized as their children for purposes of inheritance and receipt of Social Security benefits. Even though DNA testing could prove the biological connection with certainty, state statutes on paternity and on intestate succession limit the situations in which children of deceased individuals receive legal recognition. Paternity laws consider the husband to be the father of children born to his wife, but a dead man is not a "husband" under such statutes. In some states, probate laws provide that posthumous children can inherit under intestate succession if they are born within a certain number of days of their father's death. For example, New Jersey law presumes a man to be a biological (and thus legal) father to his wife's child if the child is born within 300 days after the man's death (N.J. Stat. Ann. 9:17-43[a][1]). But women who are inseminated with the deceased's sperm months or years after his death fall outside those laws. Posthumous reproduction raises questions of legal parentage, inheritance, Social Security benefits, and whether a child conceived posthumously could assert a wrongful death claim regarding his or her deceased progenitor (Shah 1996).

Courts differ in their assessment of the weight that should be given to a genetic test showing that the deceased was the biological father of a posthumously conceived child. This issue has arisen in judicial analyses about whether the child should be considered an offspring for intestate succession purposes and whether such a child should be entitled to Social Security benefits.

In *In re Estate of William Kolacy* (2000), the decedent had stored sperm before undergoing chemotherapy. A year after his death, his widow used that sperm to create twins using in vitro fertilization. His widow was denied Social Security benefits for the twins. Because the federal Social Security Act allows children to collect benefits if they could have inherited under the state's intestate succession laws, the widow brought suit to establish the children's status under state law. The court said that, although legislatures should address these issues, "We judges cannot simply put those problems on hold in the hopes that some day (which may never come) the legislature will deal with the problem in question." The court held that, once it is established that the child is the biological offspring of a decedent, the court should consider the child an heir for intestate succession purposes "unless doing so would unfairly intrude on the rights of other persons or would cause serious problems in terms of the orderly administration of estates." On the latter point, the court noted that posthumous conception could tie up estates for years. The court suggested that it would be constitutional for the legislature to impose a time limit after death for posthumous inheritance: only children born during this time would be able to inherit.

A similar result was reached by the Massachusetts Supreme Judicial Court in a decision that articulated the values that should guide decisions about inheritance in the case of posthumous conception. The court in *Woodward v. Commissioner of Social Security* (2002) highlighted "the best interests of children, the State's interest in the orderly administration of estates, and the reproductive rights of the genetic parent." As to the posthumous child's interests, the court assumed that the child should be entitled to the same protection as children conceived before a man's death. One of the state's interests could be satisfied by DNA paternity testing showing certainty of filiation. But, the court said, the state also had an interest in closure, so lawmakers should establish time limitations for posthumous claims. The court also emphasized the need for assuring reproductive rights through evidence that the man intended his sperm to be used for reproductive purposes after his death. The court remanded the case for a determination of whether the man consented to such use.

In *Woodward*, the Massachusetts Supreme Judicial Court ruled that a posthumously conceived child may be entitled to inherit under the state's intestacy laws if the following are established: (1) there is a genetic relationship between the child and the decedent; (2) the decedent affirmatively consented to creating a child after death; and (3) the decedent affirmatively consented to the support of any resulting child. The court cautioned that, even if the above criteria were met, time limitations in relation to the orderly administration of estates could prevent a claim on behalf of a posthumously conceived child.

The differences in state laws regarding paternity will lead to different outcomes for posthumous children seeking Social Security benefits. A child conceived posthumously by means of reproductive technologies will most likely not be entitled to Social Security survivor's benefits in Arizona, whereas an award of benefits is at least a possibility in Massachusetts. In an Arizona case, a woman became pregnant using in vitro fertilization with her deceased husband's sperm ten months after her husband's death and gave birth to twins, a girl and a boy. When she was denied Social Security survivor's benefits on behalf of her children, she filed suit (*Gillett-Netting v. Barnhart* 2002). Despite evidence of the husband's intent to create children after his death, the court ruled that, because the twins were not alive or "in gestation" at the time of the husband's death, they would not be entitled to inherit under Arizona's intestacy laws, and further noted that the intent of the decedent was not a factor to consider. The court also ruled that, because the twins were not in existence at the time of the husband's death, they could not demonstrate actual dependency, and because they were not considered his heirs under the intestacy laws of Arizona, they could not show presumed dependency, which is required to establish a right to Social Security benefits under federal law.

The Arizona court distinguished the Massachusetts decision in *Woodward* based on differences between the intestate statutes of the two states, noting that Massachusetts has a provision in its statutes that is absent in Arizona: "posthumous children shall be considered living at the death of their parent"

(*Gillett-Netting v. Barnhart* 2002). The court seemed to reason that Massachusetts could have defined or placed a time limitation on posthumous children but chose not to, leaving the door open to interpretation. The court noted that Arizona, unlike Massachusetts, has a specific provision for after-born heirs that requires a child to be "in gestation" in order for the child to be considered an heir. The court addressed the equal protection claim by reasoning that children created by in vitro fertilization were not treated differently under Arizona's intestacy laws because of their mode of conception but rather because they were not born or "in gestation" at the time of the decedent's death. The court further ruled that it was rational for the Social Security Administration to look to state intestate laws to determine dependency.

The Massachusetts Supreme Judicial Court in *Woodward,* like so many courts dealing with reproductive technologies, called on legislators to create a framework for deciding parenthood issues in the context of reproductive technologies: "The questions present in this case cry out for lengthy, careful examination outside the adversary process, which can only address the specific circumstances of each controversy that presents itself. They demand a comprehensive response reflecting the considered will of the people."

State legislatures have begun addressing the issue of posthumous conception. In North Dakota, "a person who dies before conception using that person's sperm or egg is not a parent of any resulting child born of the conception" (N.D. Cent. Code § 14-18-04[2]). However, in Texas, the man's paternity is recognized if the procedure is done with advance permission. The Texas statute reads, "If a spouse dies before the placement of eggs, sperm, or embryos, the deceased spouse is not a parent of the resulting child unless the deceased spouse consented in a record that if assisted reproduction were to occur after death the deceased spouse would be parent of the child" (Tex. Fam. Code § 160.707).

In Virginia, any child conceived by a married couple with the wife's egg and the consenting husband's sperm is considered to be the child of the couple, regardless of whether either party died during the ten-month period preceding the child's birth. However, if one of the genetic parents dies before implantation of an embryo, whether the embryo is created with that person's spouse or not, the deceased is considered a legal parent only if implantation occurred before the death could be reasonably communicated to the physician performing the procedure or if the deceased left written consent to be a parent before the implantation (Va. Stat. § 20-158B).

The Values Underlying the Assignment of Parentage in the Context of Reproductive Technologies

As with traditional reproduction, the goal of many of the statutes and cases governing parenthood in the context of reproductive technology is to ensure the financial support of children by providing clear indications of who the legal parents are when multiple candidates are available. This is important, given that, on the one hand, all the parties might seek parenthood, or on the other hand, all might try to foist parenthood off on one of the other candidates. The cases and statutes also provide protections for parent-child bonds once they are established—for example, by recognizing the right of a social father after a divorce to stay involved with a child created with donor sperm. They also value deliberate action, with an assumption that people who choose to be parents may indeed be "better" parents (Schultz 1990).

The emerging legal precedents in this area focus on deliberate intentional acts to create a child and to be responsible for that child. Even in situations in which the genetic parents are given the status of legal parents (such as when a couple's embryo is implanted in a surrogate gestational mother), the rationale for the result is based not on biology but on preconception intent.

Conclusion

The role of genetic testing in determining legal parenthood is in flux. In the context of third-party assisted reproduction, DNA testing is largely irrelevant because, under statutes and court rulings, assignment of legal parenthood is generally not dependent on genetic ties. However, in the context of sexual reproduction, social institutions such as genetics laboratories and courts rush to apply DNA paternity tests without sufficient consideration of the implications of such testing. This is particularly troubling in situations of private use of DNA testing by putative fathers without the mother's knowledge or consent, exhumation of bodies for paternity testing, and DNA testing of the blood relatives of deceased putative fathers. As with the various means of socially assigning parenthood in previous generations, the role of genetic testing should be determined not with reference to the ease of the testing procedure itself but rather with consideration of the social values society wants to promote.

BIBLIOGRAPHY

Adoption of Matthew B. 1991. 284 Cal. Rptr. 18. (Cal. Ct. App.).

Anderlik, M. R., and M. A. Rothstein. 2003. Assessing the quality of DNA-based parentage testing: Preliminary findings from laboratory survey. *Jurimetrics Journal* 43: 291–314.

Andrews, L. 1984. Yours, mine, and theirs. *Psychology Today* 18:20.

Clark, C. 2003. Deploying local Marine preparing for posterity: Man leaving sperm behind in cryobank. *San Diego Union-Tribune,* 3 February.

Cruzan v. Director, Missouri Department of Health. 1990. 497 U.S. 261, 278.

Curran v. Bosze. 1990. 566 N.E.2d 1319 (Ill.).

Estate of Sanders. 1992. 3 Cal. Rptr. 2d 536 (Cal. Ct. App.).

Gillett-Netting v. Barnhart. 2002. 231 F.Supp.2d 961 (D. Ariz.).

Griswold v. Connecticut. 1965. 381 U.S. 479.

In re Baby M. 1988a. 537 A.2d 1227, 1260–61 (N.J.).

In re Baby M. 1988b. 542 A.2d 52, 55 (N.J. Super. Ct.).

In re Estate of Rogers. 1990. 583 A.2d 782, 784 (N.J. Super. Ct.).

In re Estate of William Kolacy. 2000. 753 A.2d 1257 (N.J. Super. Ct.).

In re Marriage of Buzzanca. 1998. 72 Cal. Rptr. 2d 280 (Cal. Ct. App.).

In re Moschetta. 1994. 30 Cal. Rptr. 2d 893 (Cal. Ct. App.).

Jhordan C. v. Mary K. 1986. 224 Cal. Rptr. 530 (Cal. Ct. App.).

Johnson v. Calvert. 1993. 19 Cal. Rptr. 2d 494, 500 (Cal.).

Jones v. Murray. 1992. 962 F.2d 302 (4th Cir.).

Lach v. Welch. 1997. 1997 WL 536330 (Conn. Super. Ct.).

Leckie v. Voorhies. 1994. 875 P.2d 521 (Or. Ct. App.).

Lehr v. Robertson. 1983. 463 U.S. 248.

Mayfield v. Dalton. 1995. 901 F.Supp. 300, 303 (D. Haw.).

McIntyre v. Crouch. 1989. 780 P.2d 239, 245 (Or. Ct. App).

Miscovich v. Miscovich. 1997. 688 A.2d 726 (Pa. Super. Ct.).

N.A.H. v. S.L.S. 2000. 9 P.3d 354 (Colo.).

Newbart, D. 2003. UIC sperm bank gives soldiers a break. *Chicago Sun-Times,* 12 February.

Office for Protection from Research Risks. 1993. *Protecting Human Research Subjects: Institutional Review Board Guidebook,* 5–45. Bethesda, MD: National Institutes of Health.

People v. Sorensen. 1968. 437 P.2d 495 (Cal.).

Rushford v. Caines. 2001. 2001 WL 310006 (Ohio Ct. App).

S.C.G. v. J.G.Y. 2000. 2000 WL 1273472 (Ala. Ct. Civ. App).

Schultz, M. 1990. Reproductive technology and intent-based parenthood: An opportunity for gender neutrality. *Wisconsin Law Review* 1990:297–398.

Shah, M. 1996. Modern reproductive technologies: Legal issues concerning cryopreservation and posthumous conception. *Journal of Legal Medicine* 12:547.

Sudwischer v. Estate of Hoffpauir. 1991. 589 So.2d 474 (La), *cert. denied sub nom., Estate of Hoffpauir v. Sudwischer,* 504 U.S. 909 (1992).

Sutton, S. 1999. The real sexual revolution: Posthumously conceived children. *St. John's Law Review* 73:857.

Syrkowski v. Appleyard. 1983. 333 N.W.2d 90 (Mich. Ct. App.).

Syrkowski v. Appleyard. 1985. 362 N.W.2d 211 (Mich.).

Tandra S. v. Tyrone W. 1994. 648 A.2d 439, 445 (Md.).

Tyrone W. v. Danielle R. 1999. 741 A.2d 553 (Md. Ct. App.).

Union Pacific Ry. Co. v. Botsford. 1891. 141 U.S. 250.

Whalen v. Roe. 1977. 429 U.S. 589.

William M. v. Superior Court. 1990. 275 Cal. Rptr. 103 (Cal. Ct. App.).

Wise v. Fryar. 2001. 49 S.W.3d 450 (Tex. Ct. App.).

Woodward v. Commissioner of Social Security. 2002. 760 N.E.2d 257, 272 (Mass.).

CHAPTER TWELVE

Translating Values and Interests into the Law of Parentage Determination

Mark A. Rothstein, J.D.

As long demonstrated by the formal and informal adoption of children, and as more recently demonstrated by reproduction through donor gametes, genetic relatedness is not coextensive with parentage. Yet genetic ties are widely viewed by society and the courts as having a vital role in parentage that should not be disregarded lightly. The contributors to this volume have explored the ethical, legal, and social implications of parentage determinations in the light of increasingly available and sophisticated genetic testing. Here, I draw on the chapters and other sources in providing a synthesis and some recommendations.

Among the many factors complicating the analysis of genetic testing for parentage is the asymmetry between biological and social determinants of parentage. Establishing biological connections is seductively precise and now relatively simple to do; discerning the contours of relationships is frustratingly vague as a standard and notoriously difficult to do. In addition, for many of the seemingly endless variations of factual situations surrounding family relationships and parentage, predictability of outcome and flexibility in considering particular circumstances are not mutually attainable goals for the law. In other words, it is often impossible to reconcile a strict rule-based approach with a variable context-based approach to the law of parentage. The American Law Institute's (ALI) *Principles of the Law of Family Dissolution* (2002, chap. 2) refers to this tension as predictability versus individualization.

It is not my intent, or the intent of this volume, to set forth a comprehensive legal structure for determining parentage and regulating the use of genetic testing. Instead, the contributors have presented a multidisciplinary analysis of the issues intended to enrich and inform the debate over appropriate policies. I attempt here to build on the framework already developed by the Uniform Parentage Act (UPA) of 2000, as amended, and other sources to propose additional measures designed to translate societal values and interests into the law of parentage determination.

Values and Interests

The Problems

The contributors to this volume have discussed many of the complexities in parentage determinations, including (1) lack of emotionally stable and financially secure loving relationships for children; (2) deceit and distrust among men and women who seek or would be assigned the title of mothers and fathers; and (3) widespread efforts to manipulate the system for determining the rights and responsibilities of parentage, thereby invoking the alliterative notions of malicious moms and mistreated moms, deadbeat dads and duped dads.

Advances in DNA parentage testing add another layer of complexity to these problems. Although virtually definitive testing is now available, the testing process itself has the potential to undermine relationships, as described by Dan Wulff (chapter 5). The legal significance of DNA testing differs among the states, depending on various factors, such as when the testing was performed. There also has been a proliferation of surreptitious testing, usually involving testing without the knowledge or consent of the custodial mother, but sometimes testing without the knowledge or consent of the presumed father. Much of this controversial testing is performed by unregulated laboratories that are unconstrained by requirements of quality assurance and accuracy.

The difficulty in resolving these issues suggests the need to go back to first principles. What are we trying to accomplish in parentage determination? How can such decisions support rather than undermine social policy? What are the societal values and the interests of the parties implicated by the use of genetic determinations of parenthood?

The Values

Values are those aspects of social life that members of a group consider to be of intrinsic worth. Various social institutions, including the law, are structured and operated to promote the values of a society. The philosophy of law, or jurisprudence, long has pondered the connection between law and societal values. It has attempted to discern whether there are certain principal values that the law strives to embody. According to at least one formulation, freedom, responsibility, and equality are the touchstone values of the law (Bayles 1987, 350). These values, especially responsibility and equality, also are at the heart of an appropriate legal system dealing with parentage determinations.

In chapter 2, Thomas Murray suggests that the family unit should be the focus in formulating rules about parentage. The family unit is central to all the values to be advanced in parentage law. These values include encouraging marriage and the stability of marriage, truthfulness and fidelity, certainty and stability in parental relationships, and parental responsibility for child support and nurture.

The Interests

Constructing social policy to further the values mentioned above would be much easier if fewer parties had an interest in the outcome of parentage determinations and if the interests of those parties did not so frequently clash. Although it is tempting to view the interests at stake as being only those of the child, mother, and father (or fathers), there are other interests to consider. These include siblings, grandparents, government child support agencies, and even the commercial interests of laboratories performing parentage testing. There are also broader societal interests, such as preventing domestic violence.

The most frequently invoked interest is the best interest of the child, but this becomes little more than a slogan without context, as noted by Elizabeth Bartholet (chapter 8) and Michael Grossberg (chapter 7). Do the best interests of the child mean children in general? If so, does this suggest that considerations of the best interests of the child should influence the development of legislative rules rather than focus on the best interests of the particular child in each individual determination? Does the best-interests-of-the-child standard equally promote the interests of mothers and fathers? Do the best interests of the child change over the course of time and, if so, how and at what age or stage of the child's development? Do the best interests of the child, while ostensibly promoting flexibility, invariably create unpredictability in parentage determination?

Jeffrey Blustein has described the three sets of competing interests in parentage as follows. First, children require a stable, care-giving relationship that provides emotional and financial support and legal protection. Second, adults may want to raise a child for various reasons, but they also may have interests and commitments with which child rearing conflicts. Third, society at large has an interest in seeing children become well-adjusted, responsible adults (Blustein 1982, 139–56).

In chapter 4, Diane Scott-Jones focuses on the child's interests. According to her, the best interests of the child should focus on the following three factors: financial support, maintaining positive relationships, and protecting the availability of genetic knowledge if the child wants this information at the time of majority or at the time of illness. One must keep in mind that people will disagree about what is in the best interests of the child. Moreover, even though the best interest of the child is the most important interest, it is not the only interest.

The Role of Biology

In attempting to reconcile the values and interests discussed above, the fundamental issue is the degree to which social and legal conceptions of parentage are determined by genetic ties. Without resolving this overarching issue, it will be impossible to develop any consistent and principled approach to making legal determinations of parentage.

The argument has been made, based on evolutionary psychology and sociobiology, that biological relationships should be given controlling weight in determining parentage, because genetic relatedness is, from an evolutionary perspective, the sine qua non of parentage. Evolutionary theory, however, also predicts that a male would attempt to kill the children fathered by other males with the same female so that only his offspring survive and reproduce (Jones 1997). There is evidence of this phenomenon in other species (Hrdy 1979). Nevertheless, even if one can posit an evolutionary explanation for past human behavior or the current behavior of other species, it does not necessarily mean that the explanation should have any relevance for modern society or law. The greatest evolutionary advantage of *Homo sapiens* was the growth of a larynx and large brain capable of developing language and culture, including laws that set limits on the power of stronger individuals over weaker ones: "While sociobiology is thus useful for understanding the evolutionary context of human social behavior, this approach still shouldn't be pushed too far. The goal of all human activity can't be reduced to the leaving of descendants. Once human culture was firmly in place, it acquired new goals" (Diamond 1992, 98).

Even Richard Dawkins, whose writings helped popularize sociobiology, recognizes the limits of genetic explanations of human behavior: "Adoption and contraception, like reading, mathematics, and stress-induced illness, are products of an animal that is living in an environment radically different from the one in which its genes were naturally selected. The question, about the adaptive significance of behaviour in an artificial world, should never have been put; and although a silly question may deserve a silly answer, it is wiser to give no answer at all and to explain why" (Dawkins 1999, 36).

Another argument in favor of a greater role for biology in determining parentage is that increased reliance on biology (i.e., genetic testing) will restore more of a balance to parentage law, which allegedly now discounts the interests of "duped dads" in their struggles with "duplicitous, unfaithful moms" (Tesser 2002). It would be erroneous, however, to equate purely biological notions of parentage with the interests of men. Although a greater reliance on biology may help legally presumed fathers with no genetic ties to a child win disestablishment suits, the exclusive use of biology in parentage determination would interfere with the interests of legally presumed fathers in suits to establish paternity brought by men who turn out to be the biological father of a child. Thus a greater reliance on biology will advantage some men and disadvantage other men, depending on how the evidence of genetic relatedness or lack of relatedness is used.

An emphasis on biological connection also represents an adult view of parenthood: "For the child, the physical realities of his conception and birth are not the direct cause of his emotional attachment. This attachment results from day-to-day attention to his needs for physical care, nourishment, comfort, affection, and stimulation" (Goldstein, Freud, and Solnit 1973, 17). Accordingly, an excessive focus on biological ties may not necessarily promote the best interests of children.

Concerns about the proper role of biological connections in parentage lead directly to the use of DNA tests, including issues of when and by whom DNA paternity testing can be undertaken and the legal significance to be accorded the results. Those in favor of more widespread use of and weight for DNA testing argue that DNA testing establishes the certainty of biological relationships, promotes finality and financial responsibility, and supports fidelity. Those opposed to increased use of DNA testing argue that it overemphasizes the significance of biological relationships, discourages nurturing by social fathers, and promotes uncertainty in social relationships because of the possibility of later determinations of nonpaternity.

In chapter 10, Mary Anderlik Majumder proposes a four-part framework for analyzing the role of biology in parentage, which she terms biological imperative, biological presumption, biological relevance, and biological indifference. As she observes, current laws generally follow one of the two middle positions, either biological presumption or biological relevance. There has been increasing pressure, however, in the legislatures, courts, and media to give biology, and specifically the results of DNA tests, greater weight in deciding parentage.

The Law

State Parentage Law

The law of every state except Louisiana (which is civil law based) traces its parentage law to two common law doctrines: (1) the marital presumption and (2) the formal adjudication of paternity. The states have struggled with the proper approach to modernize their paternity laws and move away from these doctrines, with the results varying more now than at any time in the history of the United States, as noted by Grossberg (chapter 7).

The marital presumption, dating back to eighteenth-century England, provided that a child born to a married couple was presumed to be the child of the couple. Lord Mansfield's Rule, enunciated in 1777, added the evidentiary rule that the marital presumption could be rebutted only by proving that the husband did not have access to his wife during the period of conception (Shapiro, Reifler, and Psome 1992–93, 13–18). The presumption was based not on the needs of children "but on society's need for stability and certainty in family relationships at a time when property, and therefore often a family's livelihood, was dependent on clear rules concerning patrilineal succession" (Glennon 2000, 563).

In its earliest form, the marital presumption could be rebutted only by the testimony of the husband, but by the late nineteenth century in the United States, the evidentiary restrictions had been loosened to permit the testimony of the wife about lack of access and, in some states, evidence of sterility or impotence. The justification for the presumption also was changing to include supporting the institution of marriage, protecting the inheritance rights of children, and preventing the stigmatization of nonmarital children. The Uniform Parentage Act of 1973, while generally following the marital presumption, also permitted the child, mother, and presumed father to bring legal actions to establish or disestablish the paternity of the presumptive father. Judicial challenges dealing with the marital presumption have involved various scenarios, including the self-proclaimed biological father seeking to assert paternity, the legally presumed father seeking to deny paternity during or following divorce from the mother, and the mother seeking to deny the presumed father's paternity during or following divorce (Glennon 2000, 571–86). In many of these cases, the issue for the courts was the extent to which biological ties should dictate legal paternity.

At the same time that the marital presumption governed parentage issues for children born within a marriage, the paternity of a child born outside marriage could be established only through the courts (Roberts 1996). Because nonmarital paternity was evidence of the crime of adultery or fornication, a paternity case (originally called a "bastardy proceeding") was a quasi-criminal proceeding, with a jury trial and a burden of proof of "beyond a reasonable doubt." Over time, paternity cases involving nonmarital children became civil cases, and voluntary acknowledgments have been accorded the weight of judicial determinations (National Women's Law Center 2000, 3).

The policies underlying paternity determinations involving nonmarital children do not include supporting marital stability. The best-interests-of-the-child standard, as well as other equitable considerations, increasingly became the focus for courts attempting to decide a child's legal paternity. In doing so, the courts in nonmarital cases were faced with the same dilemma as in the marital cases of deciding how much weight should be given to biological connections.

Personal Responsibility and Work Opportunity Reconciliation Act of 1996

The Personal Responsibility and Work Opportunity Reconciliation Act of 1996 (PRWORA) made major changes in the federally supported welfare system (Public Law 104-193, 42 U.S.C. §§ 666 et seq.). The PRWORA replaced the Aid to Families with Dependent Children (AFDC) program with Temporary Assistance for Needy Families. Among other things, the PRWORA set time limits on welfare benefits (maximum of sixty weeks), imposed work requirements for recipients (failure to seek or accept work leads to disqualification), and added other restrictions on recipients receiving benefits (e.g., mandating school attendance and immunizations for children). The PRWORA also placed a high priority on collecting child support payments from noncustodial parents.

The child support provisions of the PRWORA have been criticized for setting a single standard for the obligation of nonresident fathers to pay child support. "Just because nonresident fathers as a whole can afford to pay substantially more child support than they currently pay does not mean that the fathers of children on welfare can afford to pay substantially more" (Garfinkel et al. 1999, 331). In order to collect child support from fathers of any income level, it is necessary to identify the fathers, and the PRWORA addresses this issue in detail.

The PRWORA made at least five major changes in the law of establishing paternity for purposes of welfare (National Women's Law Center 2000, 4–6). First, states must encourage voluntary paternity establishment by recognizing a signed acknowledgment of paternity as a legal finding of paternity, unless it is rescinded within sixty days. After sixty days, acknowledgments may be challenged only for fraud, duress, or material mistake of fact. States must also require that paternity is formally established before the name of an unmarried father is recorded on a birth certificate. States also must make voluntary acknowledgment widely available at birth records agencies and public and private hospitals.

Second, states must adopt laws that simplify establishing paternity in contested cases. Child support agencies must be given authority to order genetic testing without applying for a court order, the results must be readily admitted into evidence, and states must pay for the test—although they are permitted to recoup the cost from parents under certain circumstances. States also must eliminate jury trials in paternity cases and enter temporary support orders pending outcome of a paternity determination when there is clear and convincing evidence of paternity.

Third, states must give putative fathers an opportunity to bring an action to establish paternity.

Fourth, states must establish more severe consequences for failure to assist in establishing paternity than were in effect under the prior federal program. Under AFDC, applicants and recipients who failed to cooperate in establishing paternity or collecting support were sanctioned by loss of the caretaker's portion of the payment, but payments to children were unaffected. Under the PRWORA, states must reduce the payment to the family by at least 25 percent for noncooperation and may terminate the grant entirely if they choose. More than half the states now authorize termination (Turetsky 1998). A majority of states also require all child support payments by noncustodial parents to go entirely to the state, rather than a dollar amount or percentage of the payments going to increase the level of support to the family, as was permitted under AFDC. In the first year of operation of the new law, FY 1997, the amount of support money given to families receiving welfare decreased from $337 million under AFDC to $40 million under the PRWORA (Office of Child Support Enforcement 1999, table 16).

Fifth, the PRWORA pressured states to increase the number and percentage of paternities established in relation to nonmarital births to 90 percent. States failing to meet this figure may be penalized; the percentage of paternities established also affects the availability of federal incentive payments to the states.

The PRWORA famously attempted "to end welfare as we know it." For better or worse, it also ended the practice of paternity establishment as we knew it. States reacted to the new federal mandates by amending their welfare and family laws and enacting new provisions dealing with establishing paternity. Many of these changes in family law are reflected in the Uniform Parentage Act of 2000, discussed below. Viewed most sympathetically, the PRWORA replaced a failed, permissive welfare system with a system of "tough love" incentives to encourage the responsibility and self-sufficiency needed to end the cycle of dependence of "welfare families." Viewed most critically, the PRWORA is a punitive system designed to minimize governmental expenditures, enacted without regard for the best interests of children or families. Regardless of one's view of the PRWORA, any significant revisions of the law of parentage now must be reflected in both federal and state statutes.

Law Reform

The Uniform Parentage Act of 2000

The widely disparate state laws on parentage have developed despite nearly a century of efforts by the National Conference of Commissioners on Uniform State Laws to establish some degree of uniformity. The National Conference was organized in 1892 with the goal of promoting uniformity in certain state laws. Originally containing representatives from seven states, by 1912 the conference had uniform law commissioners appointed by every state. One of the first accomplishments of the conference, in 1922, was development of a Uniform Illegitimacy Act. Of the numerous other uniform acts developed by the National Conference, several of them dealt with issues related to parentage, including blood testing to determine parentage (1952), paternity (1960), and probate (1969). The Uniform Parentage Act of 1973 established, among other things, the equality of all children without regard to the marital status of their parents. It also rejected the continued use of the term *illegitimate* in favor of *child with no presumed father.* As of December 2000, nineteen states had enacted the Uniform Parentage Act of 1973 in whole, and many others had adopted it in part.

Parentage law continued to be a source of new model laws by the commissioners after the act of 1973. To deal with the rights of fathers after a mother relinquishes a child for adoption, the National Conference adopted the Uniform Putative and Unknown Fathers Act of 1988. The same year it also adopted the Uniform Status of Children of Assisted Conception Act. In 2000, the conference approved the comprehensive Uniform Parentage Act of 2000 (UPA). With the adoption of this act, the conference withdrew all the earlier uniform acts related to parentage. In December 2002, the conference adopted several amendments to the UPA, most of which were intended to make it more difficult to disestablish the rights and duties of nonmarital fathers. As of early 2005, only Delaware, Texas, Washington, and Wyoming had enacted the UPA, but enactment of uniform acts often takes several legislative sessions.

The Uniform Parentage Act of 2000 provides an excellent starting point for considering legislative strategies for dealing with determining parentage. Three articles of the UPA are particularly relevant to the issue of parentage: voluntary acknowledgment of paternity (article 3), genetic testing (article 5), and adjudication of parentage (article 6). A separate provision (article 7) deals with assisted reproduction.

Voluntary acknowledgment of paternity. As discussed above, the federal PRWORA of 1996 conditioned receipt of federal child support enforcement funds on a state's enacting laws that strengthen the effect of a man's voluntary acknowledgment of paternity. Thus a valid, unrescinded, unchallenged acknowledgment of paternity is considered equivalent to a judicial determination of paternity.

Section 302 of the UPA details the requirements for an acknowledgment of paternity. The acknowledgment must be signed (under penalty of perjury); state that the child does not have a presumed father (or has a presumed father who has signed a denial of paternity); state whether there has been genetic testing and, if so, whether the test is consistent with the claim of paternity; and state that the signatories understand that the acknowledgment is equivalent to a judicial adjudication of paternity.

Section 303 provides that a presumed father (defined in section 102[17] as a man who, by operation of law, is recognized as the father of a child until that status is rebutted or confirmed in a judicial proceeding) may sign a denial of paternity. If accompanied by an acknowledgment of paternity, the denial of paternity is equivalent to an adjudication of nonpaternity and discharges the rights and duties of the presumed father. Section 304 provides that an acknowledgment and denial of paternity may be contained in a single document and may be executed before or after the birth of a child.

Section 307 provides that a signatory may rescind an acknowledgment or denial of paternity by commencing a proceeding to do so before the earlier of sixty days after the effective date of the acknowledgment or denial or the date of the first hearing to adjudicate an issue related to the child, including a proceeding to establish support. Pursuant to section 308, after the period for rescission set forth in section 307 has expired, a signatory of an acknowledgment or denial of paternity may bring a proceeding to challenge the acknowledgment or denial only "(1) on the basis of fraud, duress, or material mistake of fact; and (2) within two years after the acknowledgment or denial is filed with the [agency maintaining birth records]."

Genetic testing. Article 5 applies to genetic testing to determine parentage undertaken voluntarily or pursuant to a court order. A court may order genetic testing if there is a reasonable dispute as to the parentage of a child. Section 503 provides that testing must be of a type reasonably relied on by experts in the field of genetic testing and must be performed in a laboratory accredited by the American Association of Blood Banks (AABB), the American Society for Histocompatibility and Immunogenetics, or an accrediting body designated by the U.S. Secretary of Health and Human Services.

Section 504 provides that the testing laboratory may establish a reliable chain of custody by documenting the names and photographs of the individuals whose biological specimens are taken, the names of the individuals who collected the specimens, the places and dates the specimens were collected, the names of the individuals who received the specimens in the testing laboratory, and the dates the specimens were received.

Section 505 provides that a man is rebuttably identified as the father of a child if the man has at least a 99 percent probability of paternity, using a prior probability of 0.50, as calculated by using the combined paternity index obtained in the testing and a combined paternity index of at least 100 to 1.

Adjudication of parentage. Article 6 sets out the substantive and procedural rules for adjudicating parentage. The UPA draws an important distinction between the applicable rules for children with a presumed father and for those with no presumed, acknowledged, or adjudicated father. Section 607 provides that a proceeding to adjudicate the parentage of a child having a presumed father, brought by a presumed father, the mother, or another individual, must be brought within two years of the birth of the child. A proceeding seeking to disprove the father-child relationship between a child and the child's presumed father may be brought at any time, if the court determines that the presumed father and mother of the child neither cohabited nor engaged in sexual intercourse with each other during the probable time of conception and that the presumed father never openly treated the child as his own.

In contrast to the limited provisions for challenging the paternity of a child with a presumed father, section 606 provides that a proceeding to adjudicate the parentage of a child having no presumed, acknowledged, or adjudicated father may be brought at any time, even after the child becomes an adult or after an earlier proceeding to adjudicate paternity has been dismissed based on the application of a statute of limitations.

Section 608 provides that in actions brought pursuant to section 607 (proceeding to adjudicate parentage when there is a presumed father), a court may deny a motion for genetic testing of the mother, the child, and the presumed father, if the court determines that the conduct of the mother or the presumed father estops that party from denying parentage and that it would be inequitable to disprove the father-child relationship between the child and the presumed father. In determining whether to deny a motion for genetic testing, section 608 provides that the court consider the best interests of the child based on (1) the length of time between the proceeding to adjudicate parentage and the time the presumed father was placed on notice that he might not be the genetic father; (2) the length of time during which the presumed father has assumed the role of father of the child; (3) the facts surrounding the presumed father's discovery of his possible nonpaternity; (4) the nature of the relationship between the child and the presumed father; (5) the age of the child;

(6) the harm that may result to the child if the presumed paternity is successfully proved; (7) the nature of the relationship between the child and any alleged father; (8) the extent to which the passage of time reduces the chances of establishing the paternity of another man and a child support obligation in favor of the child; and (9) other factors that may affect the equities arising from the disruption of the father-child relationship between the child and the presumed father or the chance of other harm to the child.

Section 609 provides that if a child has an acknowledged or adjudicated father, a signatory to the acknowledgment or denial of paternity may seek to rescind the acknowledgment or denial or challenge the paternity of the child within two years of the date of filing the acknowledgment or denial. An individual, other than the child, who is neither a signatory to the acknowledgment of paternity nor a party to the adjudication and who seeks paternity of the child must do so within two years of the effective date of the acknowledgment or adjudication.

Beyond the Uniform Parentage Act: Policy Options and Recommendations

The Uniform Parentage Act of 2000, like other documents dealing with parentage testing, attempts to reconcile a number of conflicting individual and societal interests. Among the many provisions of the UPA discussed above, two policy choices are especially significant. First, the UPA attempts to encourage voluntary acknowledgments of paternity for children with no presumed father by streamlining and regularizing the process. In this respect, the act supports the need for states to meet the requirement of the federal PRWORA of giving greater legal effect to acknowledgments. Second, the UPA attempts to balance the interests in finality, certainty, and nurturing in parentage with the interest in giving legal primacy to biological parents. It does so by establishing a limited, two-year period in which to contest the parentage of a child with a presumed father.

As originally drafted, the presumption of paternity after two years applied only to marital children. To treat nonmarital and marital children equally, in 2002, UPA section 204(a)(5) was added, which provides that a man is presumed to be the father of a child if "for the first two years of the child's life, he resided in the same household with the child and openly held out the child as his own." Once this presumption arises, it is subject to attack only under the limited circumstances set forth in section 607 for challenging a marital presumption, and it is similarly subject to the estoppel principles of section 608.

Thus, under the UPA, biology matters, but only up to a point in time when relationships have likely been established and the interests of stability and certainty outweigh genetic ties. I later set out some possible additions to and modifications of the UPA framework.

Acknowledgments and denials. Section 302(a)(4) of the UPA provides that an acknowledgment of paternity must include a statement of whether there has been genetic testing and, if so, that the results are consistent with the claim of paternity. Presumably, individuals who are excluded from paternity on the basis of a genetic test will not sign an acknowledgment, because it would be void under section 302(b)(1). Nevertheless, the UPA provision does little to discourage individuals from signing an acknowledgment in the absence of a genetic test.

The UPA promotes acknowledgments by not requiring genetic testing, but it does so as a matter of convenience, cost saving, and public policy dictated by the PRWORA rather than as a philosophical rejection of the biological model of parentage. Indeed, the act repeatedly gives priority to biological fathers so long as they exercise their rights in a timely manner. Nevertheless, a man who has had sexual relations with a woman who is about to give or who has just given birth to a child may be subject to coercion (or more subtle but still problematic manipulation) to sign an acknowledgment. The signing of an acknowledgment in such a circumstance does not further the long-term interests of the man signing the acknowledgment or those of the child, because the paternity of the child will remain in doubt as a matter of law, with the acknowledged father having the right to rescind the acknowledgment for up to two years, and beyond two years in the event of fraud.

Governmental pressure on mothers to name and procure an acknowledgment from a putative father places the state's fiscal interest in recoupment of public assistance above the child's interest in stability. From the child's perspective, preventing the disestablishment of paternity of a social but not biological father is of greater concern than establishing such paternity, as discussed by Diane Scott-Jones (chapter 4). As long as legal notions of paternity are based, in the first instance, on genetic ties, then it is essential that the claims about paternity be consistent with actual genetic ties so that they can withstand attempts to unravel them, a point made by Jeffrey Blustein (chapter 3).

One way to add greater certainty to acknowledgments is to require that they be supported by the results of genetic testing. A man who is not the biological father of a child would then be required to adopt the child so as to establish his paternal rights. Although this may have the negative effect of discouraging some men from signing acknowledgments, it will be offset by the positive effect of an increased level of certainty in acknowledgments. It will also do away with the need for actions to rescind acknowledgments set out in section 307 of the UPA. A parallel policy option would be to require denials of paternity to be supported by the results of genetic testing. The advantage of such a change would be to establish more of an absolute bar to paternity challenges.

In *Paternity of Cheryl* (2001), a father moved to set aside a judgment of paternity more than five years after he voluntarily acknowledged paternity, when genetic tests established that he was not the child's biological father. The Supreme Judicial Court of Massachusetts vacated the probate court's reopening of the case. The man's delay in asserting his right to challenge paternity meant that the child's interests in stability and continuity of support outweighed his interests. In a footnote, the court stated that "where the State requires an unmarried woman to name her child's putative father, the department [of Transitional Assistance] should require that the parties submit to genetic testing prior to the execution of any acknowledgment of paternity or child support agreement. To do otherwise places at risk the well-being of children born out of wedlock whose fathers subsequently learn, as modern scientific methods now make possible, that they have no genetic link to their children" (746 N.E.2d 500 n. 21).

Even if genetic testing is not required as a part of an acknowledgment or denial, restrictions should be placed on the fraud exception in section 308 of the UPA. Currently, the grounds for rescission are "fraud, duress, or material mistake of fact." The lack of specificity virtually ensures that artful pleading will allow some actions to go forward. A decision of the Texas Court of Appeals is instructive on this issue. In *Wise v. Fryar* (2001), the divorced father of four children born during his marriage to the defendant sought to reopen his divorce decree on the ground that subsequent genetic testing proved he was not the father of three of the children. He asserted that his ex-wife had failed to disclose her extramarital affairs and had concealed the identity of the biological father. In denying the plaintiff's motion to reopen the decree, the court distinguished between extrinsic and intrinsic fraud. Extrinsic fraud will support a reopening of a case, because it denies a losing litigant the opportunity to fully litigate his rights or defenses at trial. Intrinsic fraud, by contrast, pertains to the matter that is considered at the trial and may be rebutted by the opposing party. In *Wise,* his ex-wife's alleged perjury was deemed to be intrinsic fraud, so it was a not a basis for reopening the divorce decree. Similar results have been reached by other courts. (*Lipscomb v. Wells* 2001). Section 308 of the UPA should incorporate similar language, thereby limiting the fraud exception to "extrinsic" matters.

Notifications to presumed fathers. One source of disputed parentage is the absent husband, which may occur when the couple is separated or when the husband is away from home for a long period of time. When a married woman has a baby, her husband is the presumed father. If the husband is absent at the time of birth or at the time the birth certificate is completed, it is not clear whether he has received notice of the birth of his presumed child. When the husband later learns of the birth, a paternity dispute might arise, with all its attendant stresses and uncertainties. One way of avoiding the problem of the absent husband not knowing in a timely manner of the birth of his presumed child is for the state to send a certified notice to the husband in every instance in which a child is born to a married woman with an absent husband (defined simply and inclusively as a husband not present at the completion of the birth certificate). The notice should inform the husband of his legal rights and responsibilities and should start the time for any action for denial of paternity that he may choose to bring. As with other notices surrounding birth and parentage determinations, these notices should be sent in a multilingual format and contain culturally appropriate language.

A related issue is the use of blank spaces on birth certificates under the designation of the father. Jeffrey Parness has suggested that this lack of information on a birth certificate might trigger an immediate inquiry by the state about the identity of the father (chapter 9). In some cases, the mother may not know the father's identity; in other cases, however, the failure to indicate an alleged father may represent a mother's desire to leave her options open for later identifying the father. Expectant and new mothers should realize that this strategy is unlikely to benefit either them or their children. Mothers should not get to choose the child's father by misrepresenting the biological father of the child. Moreover, subsequent challenges to paternity brought by a wrongfully designated father will leave the mother and child in a worse condition financially and emotionally than if the true biological father had been identified at birth.

Ex parte orders for genetic testing. One of the problems associated with the current system of parentage determination is the ease with which a single parent (including noncustodial parent) may obtain genetic testing of a child. Regardless of the legal significance afforded these tests, they have a high potential to undermine the relationships in a family. I argue below that the consent of both legal parents should be required before genetic testing is performed as a voluntary (not court-ordered) procedure.

In some situations, however, a husband and presumed father may have doubts about the paternity of a child. If he expresses these concerns to his wife and attempts to get her consent for genetic testing of the child, the marriage may be irreparably harmed, even if the test later confirms that he is the biological father. To deal with these situations, within two years of the birth of a child, a suspicious presumed father should be permitted to apply to the appropriate court for an *ex parte* order authorizing the genetic testing of the child without the consent of the mother. The court should consider the best interests of the child in deciding whether to grant such an order.

For similar reasons, within two years of the birth of a child, a suspicious mother and her consenting boyfriend also should be permitted to apply to a court for an order authorizing the genetic testing of the child without the consent of the husband.

Probability of paternity based on a genetic test. Section 505 of the UPA provides that a man is rebuttably established as the father of a child if there is a 99 percent probability of paternity. The 99 percent figure was based on the AABB's standard for confirming paternity. Although twenty-seven states have laws that create a presumption of paternity below the 99 percent probability, many independent experts believe that even the 99 percent standard is too low and that modern DNA paternity determinations using the best practices of leading laboratories require a 99.9 percent probability of paternity (Anderlik 2003).

Sanctions for false statements. The birth of a child in circumstances where the paternity is unclear or a presumed father is not likely to be the biological father places both men and women in embarrassing and stressful situations. For many of them, the seemingly easy solution may be to misrepresent the likely parentage of the child. In too many situations, however, misrepresentation increases the long-term familial, financial, and emotional disruption of the child and the family unit. Public policy must encourage truthfulness at all stages of the process of determining parentage. To prevent misstatements surrounding the parentage of children, criminal sanctions should be established for a range of untruthful acts relating to, for example, statements made on a birth certificate, acknowledgment of paternity, denial of paternity, and application for a paternity test. Similar sanctions should apply to the falsification, alteration, or unlawful disclosure of the results of a paternity test. Although many states already provide that some of these misstatements constitute perjury, few, if any, states have comprehensive systems for dealing with misstatements surrounding the process of parentage determination.

Regulating Laboratory Practices

It is impossible to separate the substantive issues of the permissible circumstances for and uses of genetic testing from the more procedural issues of the protocols of laboratories performing the testing. For example, deciding who is required to consent to test a child is both a substantive issue of the rights of custodial and noncustodial parents and a procedural issue in ensuring the regularity of sample collection. Thus, even though laboratory practices are, arguably, a subset of law reform, as discussed later in this chapter, I treat them separately here to emphasize some of the unique aspects of laboratory regulation.

Laboratory practices in DNA parentage testing have a variety of potential problems, including inadequate measures to identify sample donors, lack of consent from all parties with parental responsibility, failure to maintain a chain of custody, poor quality control, insufficient protections for confidentiality, and the absence of counseling. The general issue is how to ensure that genetic testing for parentage meets an acceptable level of quality and furthers the policy interests previously identified.

Policy makers have three main options: (1) maintain the status quo, in which accredited laboratories have modest levels of professional regulation and unaccredited laboratories are unregulated; (2) place laboratory practices under the supervision of the courts, so that only court-ordered testing is permitted and quality control is governed by statutory standards; and (3) regulate laboratories through rigorous accreditation standards and government oversight of private accreditation bodies.

Status Quo

The status quo in genetic testing for parentage is unacceptable. The laboratory performing a medical test that is technically simple and has only minor implications for one's health is extensively regulated. The laboratory performing a DNA paternity test that could destroy the bonds between husband, wife, and child is, in many instances, virtually unregulated. Parentage testing has become a large, competitive, commercial enterprise in which genetic testing for curiosity, suspicion, and legal purposes is touted on the Internet, on billboards, on tabloid television shows, and elsewhere, as described by Dorothy Nelkin (chapter 1). In 2000, accredited laboratories performed 300,626 cases of family relatedness testing, double the number of cases from 1995 (American Association of Blood Banks 2001). The number of tests performed by unaccredited laboratories is unknown.

Several organizations play a role in accrediting paternity testing laboratories. Because of the pre-DNA, serological origins of paternity testing, the American Association of Blood Banks is the accrediting organization for genetic testing in paternity. Some laboratories are accredited by the American Society for Histocompatibility and Immunogenetics, because human leukocyte antigen tests were formerly the state of the art in paternity testing. Laboratories performing genetic testing for forensic purposes are regulated by the American Society of Crime Laboratory Directors and the National Forensics Science Technology Center. Laboratories performing genetic testing for clinical purposes are regulated by the College of American Pathologists and the Centers for Medicare and Medicaid Services of the Department of Health and Human Services, pursuant to the Clinical Laboratories Improvement Amendments of 1988 (CLIA).

In most states, a laboratory performing paternity testing need not be regulated by any governmental or accrediting body—and many are not. Although the test results produced by unaccredited laboratories are generally inadmissible in paternity adjudications in court, because of chain-of-custody and other inadequacies, the results may nevertheless be the basis of a dissolution of the family unit and a protracted and disruptive divorce, paternity, or custody dispute. There are no studies on the accuracy of the results of unaccredited tests, but anecdotal evidence suggests that mistakes are not infrequent (Anderlik 2003). Indeed, even a number of CLIA-certified clinical laboratories have inadequate quality assurance records for genetic testing (McGovern et al. 1999).

Paternity testing performed in AABB-accredited laboratories has been plagued by other controversies. Commercial pressures and conflicts of interest caused by giving laboratory officials responsibility for AABB laboratory regulation have led to a relaxed atmosphere in which mail-order testing and single-parent testing are tolerated, if not condoned (Anderlik 2003). Without more extensive regulation, the accreditation standards and practices could slip even further.

Court Supervision

The most restrictive option for genetic testing for parentage is to prohibit all testing except pursuant to a court order. The active role of the courts in genetic testing would prevent many of the privacy violations, and a court's discretion in ordering the testing could be used to consider the best interests of the child. Involving the courts, however, would undoubtedly increase costs and delays. Individuals who did not want the expense, exposure, and formality of the court process might be encouraged to use "underground" and unregulated laboratories. For these reasons, the model of court involvement was rejected by the Australian Law Reform Commission (2002), whose report on the topic is one of the most detailed and thoughtful treatments of the issue.

Government Oversight of Laboratories

A combination of public and private oversight of genetic testing laboratories is likely to be the most effective and politically palatable option. The Clinical Laboratories Improvement Amendments of 1988 already regulates laboratories performing tests used in clinical practice. CLIA is enforced by the Centers for Medicare and Medicaid Services. Under CLIA, laboratories complying with equally stringent state laws are exempt from compliance with federal law. New York, one of two exempt states under CLIA, has promulgated detailed standards for paternity testing (New York State Department of Health 2000). CLIA also may utilize professional organizations to engage in accreditation activities pursuant to federal regulations. Under the CLIA model, a combination of federal, state, and private enforcement would ensure that the laboratories adhere to at least minimum federal standards for quality assurance, quality control, proficiency testing, and personnel education and training. The laboratories also would be required to follow specific measures for consent, confidentiality, and related issues, as discussed here.

Another option for regulation of laboratories performing genetic parentage testing is to enact exclusive state laws regulating laboratories, thereby delegating responsibility to the states. Although this approach has the advantage of being able to proceed in the absence of federal legislation, it would permit individuals to circumvent the law by simply going to another state for testing.

Thus, to escape a restrictive law in state *X*, the testing could be performed by a laboratory in state *Y*. State laws also could differ in the standards used for determining parentage and in other important respects. As a default approach in the absence of federal legislation, however, state enactments could help prevent shoddy and predatory laboratory practices.

Essential Elements of Laboratory Regulation

The technical aspects of laboratory standards and practices are beyond the scope of this book and the expertise of this author. Suffice it to say that whatever framework is enacted to regulate laboratories, it should include a requirement of best practices accepted by experts in the field. There are other key elements of laboratory regulation, and six of the most essential ones are discussed here.

Applicability. Currently, many laboratories, even some AABB-accredited laboratories, offer two classes of testing. One class uses the best methods and practices, which generates results admissible in judicial proceedings. Another class of testing, however, does not certify the source of sample and therefore is not admissible in court. The potential consequences of the test results, not their possible use in a legal proceeding, should determine the standards applicable to the testing. Consequently, the stringent requirements for consent, chain of custody, and other aspects of the testing should apply to all genetic testing to determine parentage.

Consent. To test a minor, in the absence of a court order, consent should be obtained from all parents with parental responsibility. Adoption of this recommendation would effectively prohibit one-parent testing by both custodial and noncustodial parents. New York State law, as well as guidelines from the United Kingdom (Department of Health 2001) and the Australian Law Reform Commission (2002), also prohibit one-parent consent for testing.

Verification of consent. Laboratories should be required to verify the identity and consent of authorized individuals by requiring the presentation of a government-issued photo identification card or through similar measures. The signed consent forms attesting to the legal authority of the individual to give consent for testing should be retained by the laboratory.

Confidentiality. Every laboratory should be required to have a confidentiality policy setting forth the measures to be taken to prevent the inadvertent disclosure of test results. All employees with access to test results should be required to undergo confidentiality training, including the methods for and importance of protecting confidentiality. Employees also should be required to sign a statement pledging to maintain confidentiality.

Counseling. Because of the significant social implications of test results, all results should be given in person. The laboratories should refer individuals to counseling services available in the community. In addition, as necessary, laboratories should advise individuals of resources for intervention in cases of domestic violence.

Sanctions. A series of stringent sanctions should be in place to enforce the regulation of genetic testing for parentage. For laboratories, the knowing and willful failure to verify authority to give consent for testing or failure to protect confidentiality of test results should be a criminal offense. In addition, as already contained in section 504 of the UPA, signing a laboratory report known to be false should be considered perjury. For individuals, it should be a criminal offense to submit false documentation to obtain a parentage test, to misrepresent parental authority over a child to authorize consent, or to alter the written report of the results of a genetic test for parentage. In addition, the nonconsensual collection of a DNA sample for analysis should be unlawful. This will eliminate the testing of napkins, straws, and other personal items without consent. The requirements also could be written to cover "fidelity testing" (Anderlik 2003).

Unresolved Issues

The recommendations in this chapter do not address all the issues needed to reform the system of parental rights and duties under law. Although some of the unresolved issues are beyond the scope of "genetic ties and the family," it is important to present a more complete agenda of items needing additional consideration.

Child Support Obligations of Nonbiological Fathers

If adopted, the recommendations would lead to greater certainty in acknowledgments and denials of paternity, notice requirements for presumed fathers, *ex parte* orders for some genetic testing, sanctions for false statements, and better regulation of paternity testing laboratories. Although calculated to bring greater fairness and accountability to parentage determinations, these recommendations do not address the central complaint of "paternity fraud victims"—the child support obligations of nonbiological fathers. Among other things, self-proclaimed paternity fraud victims and their advocates assert that it is unfair to require innocent victims of paternity fraud to support another man's child, that their payment of child support to nonbiological families often results in the impoverishment of their (new) biological families, that child support payments are not deducted from income in determining eligibility for welfare, and that court-imposed sanctions for arrearages in support obligations (e.g., suspension of driver's and professional licenses) leave them unable to earn the income needed to support both their biological and nonbiological children. Their solution to this perceived oppression is to permit DNA paternity testing at any time, to terminate support obligations on a showing of nonpaternity, and to order the recoupment of all prior child support payments from the mother. As suggested in this chapter and elsewhere in this volume, however, these blunt approaches are unlikely to promote the best interests of children.

In chapter 6, Nancy Dowd explores the connection between welfare policy and parentage policy. Undoubtedly, a comprehensive approach is needed to address these interrelated issues. Even if the reforms suggested above were enacted, the benefits would mostly be prospective. For example, future notification of presumed fathers will not help current fathers who received no such notification. Thus some transitional measures may be necessary to integrate the future reforms with current cases.

Unregulated DNA Testing

The regulatory framework for paternity testing laboratories proposed in this chapter would not affect offshore laboratories that advertise on the Internet and do their business by mail. It is unclear whether effective sanctions may be imposed against these entities, just as regulating offshore gambling and other enterprises has proved difficult. Nevertheless, the motivation to use these services would be lessened by some of the recommendations presented earlier, such as setting clear time limits for challenging paternity and permitting *ex parte* testing pursuant to a court order. In addition, laws making it a crime to collect samples for the genetic testing of children without the consent of both parents should help persuade suspicious parents that such testing is not a good idea.

Bad Faith on the Part of Parents

Despite the best efforts of legislators and judges, it is impossible to prevent all harms to children caused by parents who are mean-spirited, conniving, and concerned only with their own financial and psychic interests. Numerous scenarios can be imagined in which the system can be abused by a determined parent. Here are two examples.

A married couple has a child. The wife (but not the husband) knows or strongly suspects that the husband is not the father of the child. She says nothing until two years and one day later (after the challenge period under the UPA). She then leaves her husband and takes the child to live with her boyfriend (the father of the child), who becomes the child's social as well as biological father. Under the UPA, the ex-husband has no recourse and is obligated to pay child support. The only potential recourse would be a tort claim by the ex-husband against the ex-wife, and recovery in such a case is doubtful.

Another married couple, shortly after the birth of their first child, gets a divorce. The ex-husband has little to do with the child (just enough to prevent termination of parental rights), and he is excused from child support obligations by his ex-wife because he is impoverished. The ex-husband then uses the two-year rule of the UPA to block the social father, who has contributed financial support and nurturing, from establishing parental rights or adopting the child.

Clearly, broad reform of the parentage system is merely the first step in preventing a range of abusive practices by parents.

Conclusion

Two conflicting pressures are increasingly being brought to bear on the law of parentage. One of the pressures comes from the emergence of new families. For example, as discussed by Lori Andrews (chapter 11), the children of a family may be the result of assisted reproductive techniques, which often serve to separate the biological from the social component of parenting. Similarly, the growth in alternative families (e.g., unmarried couples, single parent, gay and lesbian couples) are challenging the prior norm of children being born and raised in a family with a married father and mother. An increase in "traditional" adoption also refutes the argument that families must be biologically linked. These new families suggest that parenting is more about relationships with children and providing children with a loving, supportive, and nurturing environment than about mere biological connection.

The countervailing pressure, often associated with public and private financial interests, is responsible for a more biological view of parentage. Federal and state welfare laws now require increased efforts to identify the biological fathers of children in an effort to recoup child support payments made by the government. Similarly, the fathers' rights movement and its legislative supporters seek to facilitate disestablishment actions in which biological evidence of nonpaternity can be used to terminate child support obligations and even recoup prior payments.

Scientific advances support both of these opposing pressures. Whereas new reproductive technologies are used to create "new families," genetic testing provides the definitive evidence to prove or disprove paternity according to the biological view of parentage. Although several recommendations have been discussed in this chapter, it is not clear whether any policies can reconcile all of these interests while promoting broad societal values. As in other domains, scientific advances, including DNA-based paternity testing, must be a means to a socially desirable end, not an end in itself.

BIBLIOGRAPHY

American Association of Blood Banks. 2001. *Parentage Testing Standards Committee, Annual Report Summary for 2000*. Bethesda, MD: The Association.

American Law Institute. 2002. *Principles of the Law of Family Dissolution*. Newark, NJ: The Institute.

Anderlik, M. R. 2003. Assessing the quality of DNA-based parentage testing: Findings from a survey of laboratories. *Jurimetrics Journal* 43:291–314.

Australian Law Reform Commission. 2002. Discussion Paper 66, Protection of Human Genetic Information 31, DNA Parentage Testing. www.austlii.edu.au/au/other/alrc/publications/dp/66/31Parentagetesting.html.

Bayles, M. D. 1987. *Principles of Law: A Normative Analysis*. Boston: D. Reidel.

Blustein, J. 1982. *Parents and Children: The Ethics of the Family*. New York: Oxford University Press.

Dawkins, R. 1999. *The Extended Phenotype: The Long Reach of the Gene*. Oxford: Oxford University Press.

Department of Health. 2001. *Code of Practice and Guidance on Genetic Paternity Testing Services*. London: The Department.

Diamond, J. 1992. *The Third Chimpanzee.* New York: Harper Collins.

Garfinkel, I., S. McClanahan, D. Meyer, and J. Seltzer. 1999. Conclusion. In *Fathers under Fire,* ed. I. Garfinkel, S. McClanahan, and D. Meyer, 333–34. New York: Russell Sage Foundation.

Glennon, T. 2000. Somebody's child: Evaluating the erosion of the marital presumption of paternity. *West Virginia Law Review* 102:547.

Goldstein, J., A. Freud, and A. J. Solnit. 1973. *Beyond the Best Interests of the Child.* New York: Free Press.

Hrdy, S. B. 1979. Infanticide among animals: A review, classification, and examination of the implications for the reproductive strategies of females. *Ethology and Sociobiology* 1:13.

Jones, O. D. 1997. Evolutionary analysis in law: An introduction and application to child abuse. *North Carolina Law Review* 75:1117.

Lipscomb v. Wells. 2001. 761 N.E.2d 218 (Ill. Ct. App.).

McGovern, M. M., M. O. Benach, S. Wallenstein, R. J. Desnick, and R. Keenlyside. 1999. Quality assurance in molecular genetic testing laboratories. *Journal of the American Medical Association* 281:835–40.

National Women's Law Center and Center on Fathers, Families and Public Policy. 2000. *Family Ties: Improving Paternity Establishment Practices and Procedures for Low-Income Mothers, Fathers and Children.* Washington, DC: The Centers.

New York State Department of Health, Clinical Laboratory Evaluation Program. 2000. Laboratory Standards. www.wadsworth.org/labcert/clep/Survey/StandardsMenu.html.

Office of Child Support Enforcement, U.S. Department of Health and Human Services. 1999. *22nd Annual Report to Congress.* Washington, DC: Government Printing Office.

Paternity of Cheryl. 2001. 746 N.E.2d 488 (Mass.).

Roberts, P. 1996. *A Guide to Establishing Paternity for Non-Marital Children: Implementing Provisions of the Personal Responsibility and Work Opportunity Reconciliation Act of 1996.* Washington, DC: Center for Law and Social Policy.

Shapiro, E. D., S. Reifler, and C. L. Psome. 1992–93. The DNA paternity test: Legislating the future paternity action. *Journal of Law and Health* 7:1.

Tesser, L. J. 2002. Dad or duped? *Family Advocate* 25(2):29–31.

Turetsky, V. 1998. *State Child Support Cooperation and Good Cause: A Preliminary Look at State Policies.* Washington, DC: Center for Law and Social Policy.

Wise v. Fryar. 2001. 49 S.W.3d 450 (Tex. Ct. App.).

Index